The 86 Healing Foods

How to Eat your Way to Perfect Health

Rachel Fontaine

The 86 Healing Foods

How to Eat your Way to Perfect Health

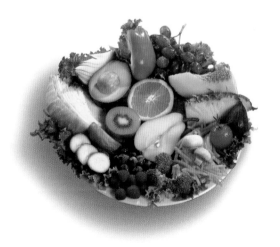

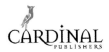

CARDINAL
PUBLISHERS

The 86 Healing Foods :
How to Eat Your Way to Perfect Health

English translation : Robert Williams, Ars Poetica Editorial Services
Copyediting : Esme Terry
Photography : Julie Léger
Cover photography : Claude Charlebois and Linda McKenty
Graphic design : Luc Sauvé
Layout : Richard Morrissette and Luc Sauvé

We acknowledge the financial support of the Government of Canada through the Book Publishing Industry Development Program (BPIDP) for our publishing activities and the support of the Government of Quebec through the tax credits for book publishing program - SODEC.

 Patrimoine canadien Canadian Heritage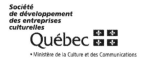

ISBN-10 : 2-920943-21-9
ISBN-13 : 978-2-920943-21-6

Cardinal Publishers/Éditions Cardinal
5400 Place de Jumonville, suite 304
Montreal, Quebec, Canada
H1M 3L7

Printed in China

A Return to Our Origins

Did you know that onions protect the blood against the dangerous effects of certain fats? Or that ginger is an effective treatment for rheumatism, arthritis and motion sickness?

Many of us know something of the healing powers of garlic, the beneficial effect of tea on digestion, the abundance of vitamins in oranges and lemons to fight colds, and the importance of a diet containing carrots and spinach: our mothers knew of the health benefits of these foods, as did their own mothers. But what about the astonishing medicinal powers of avocados, mushrooms, honey, turmeric, blueberries, parsley and cabbage?

For centuries, different cultures explored the medicinal properties of the foods they ate, to fight infections and prevent diseases. The Chinese, for example, widely used food combinations and diet to combat illness, and for this their cuisine is world renowned. The foods of several other Asian cultures developed in similar fashion, and, closer to home, the ancient Greeks and Romans would concoct fruit- and vegetable-based potions and elixirs to cure a variety of ailments.

By the end of the 20th century, nutritionists, doctors and pharmacologists, supported by the latest scientific studies, began to focus on the incredible properties of different foods and how they could act as natural medicines. Their research has been published in thousands of articles, and countless clinical studies have shown overwhelmingly positive findings as to the potent medicinal properties found in foods like broccoli, cabbage, fish, beans, green tea—and numerous other foodstuffs that can easily be incorporated into our daily meals. Yet we often ignore these encouraging findings and continue to be plagued with common, recurrent health problems. Other recent studies have made clear links between the longevity of certain groups of people and the kinds of the food they eat—almost invariably diets consisting mainly of fresh foods, with minimal processing.

These new discoveries can be discouraging to the average North American who has already embraced the convenience of industrially packaged, ready-to-eat foods. We tend to believe that the latest innovations and advances in the food industry must be working in our favor—after all, that's what the ads are telling us! But we should be aware that the vast majority of foods found in our supermarkets—often those taking up the most shelf space—are the foods with the lowest nutritional values. Most of the pre-packaged foods that we consume, while clearly marked "enriched with vitamins," are also stuffed with excessive quantities of salt, sugar, fats, coloring agents and additives: substances that, in excess, are harmful to our health and well-being. Believing that we are benefiting from the latest advances in food science, we have become disconnected from the old-fashioned, common sense values which told us that the best way to stay healthy was to choose the freshest fruits, vegetables and whole grains found in nature.

In fact, an ever-growing number of nutritionists are in agreement that we should return to our origins and consume fresh produce and products; as much to protect ourselves against disease as to remedy those health conditions that we may already suffer from. Many excellent books have been published on the subject of natural food treatments, carefully and precisely explaining studies that have been conducted on the foods that unwell people have eaten as treatments, and how, more often than not, they have returned to perfect health in ways that appear almost miraculous.

With these invaluable discoveries in mind, this book aims at something else, namely to familiarize us with the specific health benefits associated with a variety of natural foods. This book is not about listing and quoting and referencing the various studies conducted by research scientists; instead it focuses on the different roles that the natural remedies found in whole foods can play in our diet and cooking as we try to include more and more of them in our meals each day.

In the first half of the book you will find a listing of all the principal foods and food groups, each with their health benefits revealed. Included is some essential information about the specific health-giving benefits of the 86 healing foods covered here, as well as directions on how best to take advantage of their therapeutic and healing powers. Each entry offers a knowledge and understanding of that food item and highlights its qualities. Practical information is given on how to prepare these foods, as well as how to choose, store and preserve them.

The second half of the book is aimed at anyone—be they a simple food-lover or a true gourmet—who is looking to reap the health-giving rewards of these wonderful, delicious foods. Included are recipes that have been selected and adapted to bring out the best of the extraordinary health benefits of each of these ingredients. The foods used in each recipe have been chosen first and foremost for their healing properties. This does not mean that they do not also have preventive properties; on the contrary, recent studies in both Europe and North America have shown that most foods with curative properties can also protect against certain diseases. This book is therefore written as much for the person who is already in good health and is looking to maintain it, as it is written for readers afflicted with one or more health problems that they are struggling to overcome.

Start now by checking out your favorite ingredients. May it lead you on a journey to discovering the pleasures of wholesome foods while at the same time knowing that you are working to take better care of your health and well being!

Part 1

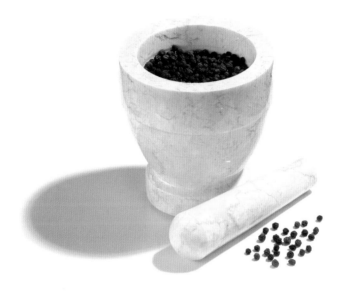

A Pharmacy in the Kitchen Cupboard

If you have health problems, it is quite likely that your doctor has recommended you eat better, regardless of the illness you suffer from. If your doctor has not already discussed your diet and eating habits with you, he or she should soon. Why? Because, according to Hippocrates, no doctor should ignore the importance of a healthy diet, since it not only has an extremely beneficial effect on your health, it can also play a part in healing a range of different ailments and diseases. Throughout history, mankind has relied on various foodstuffs to relieve illness, and in many cases it is these same foods that scientific research is now rediscovering and recognizing as extraordinary in their medicinal value: foods that can help the body fight cancer, cardiovascular disease and a host of other afflictions that compromise our quality of life. What follows is the principle of "miracle foods."

Inviting Mother Nature to the Table

Should we be astonished to learn that fresh fruits and vegetables are at the top of the list of foods that heal? Those of us who have read the Old Testament know that it was a fruit offered to Adam and Eve at the time of Creation that changed the course of history. They were punished for eating this fruit of knowledge and their legacy is supposedly our daily suffering. Does this mean that fruit—and the apple in particular—should not be eaten? Obviously not, it is quite the contrary and we all know this. Moreover, if this Bible story is to be believed, we should take note that Adam and Eve ate the forbidden fruit as a means to acquiring divinity. In this regard, we cannot completely fault them.

All **fruits**, without exception, possess fundamental nutrients that are essential to a balanced diet. Fruits are rich in vitamins, minerals, dietary fiber and energy, all of which are critically important for the proper functioning of the body and for maintaining good health. Though fruits generally contain more sugar than vegetables, fruit sugar (fructose) raises the blood sugar level at a much slower rate than does sucrose, the sugar found in white table sugar and in refined carbohydrates such as white flour. Fruit, therefore, can help to stabilize a person's energy levels, while refined sugar causes wide fluctuations in energy. A good many fruits have now been studied clinically and there is solid evidence of their antibiotic, anti-inflammatory and anti-viral therapeutic properties, as well as their ability to prevent certain types of cancer. This book takes into account these very positive conclusions, but without devoting too much space to referencing specific studies, since it is first and foremost a practical guide to everyday nutrition: a guide for people wishing to preserve and improve their health by eating a balanced diet. Naturally, if you are healthy, you will most certainly discover in this book additional benefits through eating a wider variety of fruits. A healthier, more balanced diet will play a greater preventive role and will help you preserve all aspects of your optimum physical fitness.

Vegetables, in fact, hold an even more important place in a properly balanced diet than fruits. However, since many of us have a habit of turning up our noses at vegetables, it has become a bigger hurdle for us to include more of them in our daily meals, in sufficient amounts. A great way to do this is to eat vegetables raw as an appetizer and by combining them with the fruits that we love. Because fruits are sweet, they stimulate our appetite and so we discover and experience their incredible versatility. Yet, no fruit or vegetable is in itself perfect; only by mixing them and increasing the varieties that we eat will we achieve our highest health potential.

If a green salad containing strawberries or clementines does not appeal to you, or if you would tend to decline an salad of raw beet and carrot, you may well be turning down the chance to discover a whole new universe of astonishing flavors. This sensory exploration of mixtures and flavors can help broaden your tastes and introduce you to foods you've never tried before, with benefits you were previously unaware of. The recipes in this book have been designed with the goal of helping the average person overcome his or her prejudices towards the perceived blandness of vegetables and their reputed lack of good flavor. Since it is now undeniable that vegetables are natural medicines—an almost unlimited source of prevention against a wide array of diseases and ailments—we must not forget that they can also be prepared and cooked in very little time, making savory dishes that are fit for even the most discriminating of palates.

Besides fruits and vegetables, **cereals** and grains are an essential part of our diet. They are found in our breads and cakes and, of course, our breakfast cereals. However, the colourful boxes of breakfast cereal we see in long rows at the supermarket contain, more often than not, grains that have been robbed of their health-giving properties and coated in excessive measures of sugar and chemical preservatives. It is possible to create your own flavorful blend of cereal grains that retains all the health-giving properties. Making your own breakfast cereal also has the advantage of allowing you to choose and include a wider variety of grains and ingredients, such as oats, corn, rye, flaxseed and spelt. Consider, too, the possibility—and appeal—of including grains like millet and barley as an accompaniment to a meal, in the same way we are used to doing with potatoes, rice or couscous.

Among the other foods that belong to our kitchen-shelf pharmacy, **fish** and **seaweeds** in particular should be noted, especially the so-called fatty fish, such as salmon, herring, mackerel, tuna and sardines. Add to this list **tea**, **legumes** (also known as "pulses," namely peas, beans, peanuts, alfalfa and soybeans), **tofu** and **yogurt**, and we have all we need to live in excellent health to the ripe old age of 125!

Though most forms of meat (animal protein) have been excluded from the contents of this book, it is *not* because they are considered unhealthy foods. On the contrary, in moderation, meat is highly nutritious and our emphasis on predominantly non-meat foods does not mean that meat should be avoided in a healthy diet. Meat contains the proteins our bodies need, as well as all the essential amino acids necessary for good health. It is also a rich source of minerals, trace elements and vitamins, particularly vitamin B_{12} which is involved in the production of red blood cells. However, we should bear in mind that the over-consumption of meat, especially in North America, can lead to a number of health problems and premature deaths. It is worth noting that a single serving of meat once a day is sufficient to cover most of our daily protein requirements. Moreover, a combination of foods including fish, legumes, oil seeds and a number of soy-based foods may be a healthier protein alternative to meat.

In short, if we want to adopt a healthy and healing diet, the most basic rule to follow is to increase our intake of fruits and vegetables, both in quantity and variety, and to reduce our consumption of meat, fats, refined sugar and processed foods. This does not mean that we must strictly abandon all our bad eating habits in one day; rather, we should simply begin to adopt new eating habits and, little by little, teach ourselves how to eat wisely and healthily. How do we accomplish this? First, by knowing more about the healing foods we have easy access to, and second, by taking small steps to integrate these foods into our diet by including them into our meals in imaginative and delicious ways.

What are these healing foods? What are their health-giving medical properties? Do they have dangers or negative side effects and, if so, can these be avoided while we continue to benefit from the goodness of these foods? How can we integrate these wonderful foods into our daily meals? What are the combinations of foods that enhance their curative powers? How do we store these foods and ingredients so that we can enjoy them longer? The answers to these questions follow for each of the 86 healing foods that we have compiled for you. If you think you already know these foods well, take another look through these pages before moving on to the recipes. We are ready to bet that you will learn a great deal more about these natural foods and you will discover why, quite rightly, they are considered essential for the preservation of good health.

The *86* Healing Foods

Apple

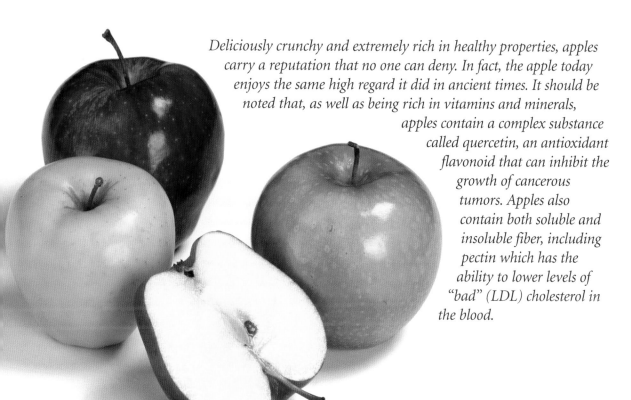

Deliciously crunchy and extremely rich in healthy properties, apples carry a reputation that no one can deny. In fact, the apple today enjoys the same high regard it did in ancient times. It should be noted that, as well as being rich in vitamins and minerals, apples contain a complex substance called quercetin, an antioxidant flavonoid that can inhibit the growth of cancerous tumors. Apples also contain both soluble and insoluble fiber, including pectin which has the ability to lower levels of "bad" (LDL) cholesterol in the blood.

Health Benefits

- Diuretic
- Effective treatment for diarrhea
- Helps prevent dental cavities
- Laxative
- Lowers blood cholesterol
- Reduces the risk of heart disease
- Revitalizes tissues

Put To Good Use

The old saying "an apple a day keeps the doctor away" is still very much true, as long as you eat your apple with the peel on, since it is there that most of the fruit's health benefits are contained.

An apple each morning on an empty stomach is one of the best cleansers and detoxifiers for the body. A small apple each evening before bed is an effective prevention against constipation. Eaten at the end of a meal, an apple not only cleans the teeth and freshens the breath, it also stimulates the gums.

Low in calories, an apple is the perfect snack for people looking to maintain their ideal weight.

Beauty Secret

Fresh apple juice applied to the face, neck, breasts and abdomen firms up tissues.

A

Caution

Particularly vulnerable to insects, apples are commonly sprayed with pesticides while they grow. Furthermore, to preserve their firmness, they are often coated in a digestible wax. If you cannot obtain organic fruit, carefully wash all apples if you choose to eat them with the peel on.

If you experience an itchy reaction in the mouth or tightness in the throat after eating apples, you may have Oral Allergy Syndrome (see entry for Orange on page 86).

Selecting & Storing

Among the many varieties of apple available on the market, some of the best for eating fresh are Melba, MacIntosh, Gala, Red and Golden Delicious, and Russet. Cortland, Spartan, Empire, Ida Red, and Rome Beauty are varieties that are just as good when eaten cooked as when eaten fresh. Apples are usually picked before they reach maturity but they can be kept for several weeks in the refrigerator.

Culinary Use

Given that it is preferable to eat apples fresh, none of their properties are lost when added to salads of lettuce, other vegetables or fruit. When cooked, they can be added to curries or stews. And of course, we can always enjoy their flavor when we turn them into applesauce, pies, tarts, turnovers, crisps and many other baked delicacies.

Recipes

- Apple, Pear and Prune Purée (page 136)
- Artichoke Apple Avocado Salad (page 216)
- Buckwheat Muffins with Apple and Beet (page 140)
- Budwig Cream (page 137)
- Cress Salad with Apple, Hazelnut and Chèvre (page 156)
- Home-Style Baked Apples (page 239)
- Hot Cider with Cinnamon (page 245)

Great Combinations

An appetizer made of lettuce, apples and walnuts combines several important nutrients: vitamin C and carotene from the lettuce, fiber and complex carbohydrates from the apples, and fatty acids, omega-3, vitamin E and fiber from the walnuts. All of these ingredients, when topped off with a simple olive oil dressing (oil, lemon and mustard), play a protective role towards the cardiovascular system.

Healthful Hints

To make a great applesauce, add the juice of half a lemon and the zest of half an orange to the apples as they are being cooked. For naturally sweetened applesauce, use figs and raisins instead of sugar; add these about 10 minutes before the end of cooking.

Good To Know

When it comes to nutrition properties, apple juice is no substitute for eating the whole, fresh fruit. However, apple juice is always preferable to any soft drink.

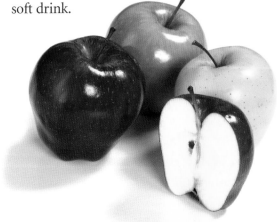

Apple Cider Vinegar

The vinegar made from apple cider has been long recognized as a treatment for a number of illnesses and infections. It contains several minerals and is rich in phosphorus and potassium. It also offers a range of medicinal properties, particularly if the vinegar is unpasteurized. Naturopaths recommend the use of apple cider vinegar for a variety of medical uses, notably to aid digestion, to treat arthritis and osteoporosis, and as a stimulant for the immune system. Its properties as an antiseptic, astringent and invigorator are well established, making it an effective home remedy for external use.

Health Benefits

- Lessens chronic fatigue
- Lowers blood pressure
- Promotes digestion
- Protects against gastroenteritis
- Relieves arthritis
- Relieves headaches brought on by indigestion
- Relieves itching due to psoriasis, diaper rash, athlete's foot, hemorrhoids, vaginitis, dandruff
- Relieves sore throat
- Stimulates appetite
- Treats kidney and bladder infections

Home Remedies

Digestion

To improve digestion, mix 1 tbsp (15 ml) apple cider vinegar with hot water and drink before each meal.

Sore throat

As soon as the first symptoms are noticed, gargle three or four times a day with a solution of 1 to 2 tbsp (15 to 30 ml) apple cider vinegar diluted in warm water.

Blocked ear

Once any build-up of earwax has been removed, put a few drops of solution made up of equal parts water and apple cider vinegar into the ear. This remedy will re-establish the acidity of the auditory canal and help stop bacterial infection.

Caution

Apple cider vinegar is not recommended for people suffering from stomach pain or ulcers, and it may provoke allergies if consumed on a regular basis. If you wish to take advantage of its health benefits, introduce it slowly and progressively into your regular diet.

It is not advisable to use vinegar to whiten teeth since its acidity creates an environment favorable to plaque-causing bacteria.

Selecting & Storing

Be sure to choose apple cider vinegar that is unfiltered and unpasteurized if you wish to take advantage of its full benefits. Like all vinegars, apple cider vinegar keeps well for long periods.

Culinary Use

Apple cider vinegar is included in many excellent salad dressings and vinaigrettes. It also heightens the flavors of cold pasta salads.

Recipes

- Blueberry Vinaigrette (page 227)
- Fresh Grape Jam (page 136)
- Super-Healthy Vinaigrette (page 227)

Beauty Secrets

Shiny hair

Mix 6 tbsp (90 ml) apple cider vinegar with 2 cups (500 ml) warm water to make a natural rinse which will enhance the hair's luster after washing.

Restores complexion

One part apple cider vinegar mixed with seven parts water makes an excellent toner for the face after washing.

Good To Know

Apple cider vinegar, of course, is made from cider, which is in turn produced from fermented apples. From the action of bacteria and yeast on the apple juice, and exposure to the air, acetic acid (vinegar) and hundreds of other compounds are produced.

A good apple cider vinegar is produced with care and patience in barrels of oak, ideally using organically or ecologically grown apples. Vinegars made from rice or wine are produced in much the same fashion.

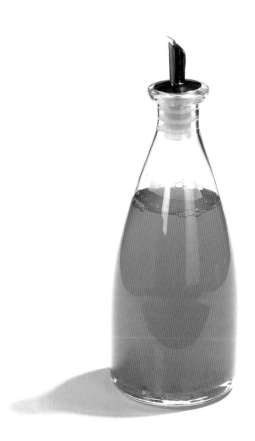

Apricot

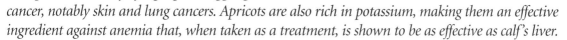

This savory, highly nutritious fruit is easily digested when consumed very ripe. It contains carotene, which accounts for the beautiful orange color of the fruit's flesh. Beta carotene, a substance found in numerous fruits and vegetables, is both an antioxidant and a stimulant for the immune system. By virtue of this combination, apricots have particular benefit for people struggling with cancer, notably skin and lung cancers. Apricots are also rich in potassium, making them an effective ingredient against anemia that, when taken as a treatment, is shown to be as effective as calf's liver.

Health Benefits

- Appetite stimulant and palate freshener
- Combats anemia
- Cures bouts of depression and insomnia
- Helps in the prevention of cancer (lung, pancreas and skin)
- Helps prevent diarrhea

Home Remedy

If you are suffering from anemia, eat four dried apricots daily before breakfast.

Caution

People who are allergic to aspirin should avoid eating apricots.

The almond-like nut contained in the pit of an apricot can cause severe illness and, if consumed in large enough amounts, intoxication.

Selecting & Storing

Choose fruit with a rich golden-orange color. Apricots with reddish hues are generally the sweetest. They can be stored, like most fruits, at room temperature until they are fully ripe, after which they should be kept in the refrigerator.

Culinary Use

To cook dried apricots, first soak them in water or fruit juice (apple or orange) until they become tender. You can add apricots to meat stews, along with nuts and other dried fruits of your choice (such as raisins or figs) that have been allowed to simmer for at least 20 minutes.

Recipes

- Apricot, Fig and Clementine Purée (page 135)
- Warm Fig and Apricot Fruit Compote (page 239)

Beauty Secret

Natural Facial Mask

Applied externally, apricots offer an excellent invigorator for the face. To obtain a softening effect, beat the flesh of a single apricot with 1 tsp (5 ml) of milk, then add 1 tsp (5 ml) of lemon juice. Leave the mask on for 15 minutes before rinsing off with warm water.

Good To Know

A fresh apricot contains fewer calories than a dried apricot. Dried apricots, however, contain much more beta carotene than the ripe, fresh fruit.

Artichoke

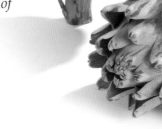

In times past, this "edible thistle" has been celebrated as an aphrodisiac. Nowadays, it is better known for stimulating digestion and lowering blood sugar. Although artichoke contains very little fat and is a good source of fiber, it is richer in sodium than most fruits and vegetables. It also contains folic acid, a nutrient that is especially important for pregnant women, as well as magnesium and potassium.

Health Benefits

- Aids in the elimination of urea and surplus cholesterol
- Helps treat Irritable Bowel Syndrome (IBS)
- Relieves problems related to digestion

Put To Good Use

The cooking water from artichokes makes an excellent stock for a vegetable soup.

Caution

Artichoke leaf extract should not be taken for obstructed bile ducts of the gall bladder. This extract stimulates bile production, which can cause serious problems. The cooking water from artichokes should not be used by people with gout, arthritis, or those suffering urinary tract infections associated with strong concentrations of minerals.

Selecting & Storing

Choose artichokes that are compact, heavy and firm, with clean, closed leaves that are a pleasing olive green color. The younger the artichoke, the more delectable the flesh. Artichokes will keep in a plastic bag in the refrigerator for about a week.

Culinary Use

Preserved artichoke hearts should always be kept on hand. They make delicious, healthy appetizers that can be prepared quickly, and they are a good complement to raw vegetables and salads. If you wish to eat the whole artichoke, it can be cooked more rapidly in the microwave (see page 149).

Recipes

- Artichoke Apple Avocado Salad (page 216)
- Artichokes with Garlic and Lemon (microwave recipe, page 149)

Healthful Hints

To prevent artichoke from discoloring, cut it with a stainless steel knife or scissors and add lemon juice to the cooking water.

Good To Know

To eat an artichoke, remove the leaves one by one, beginning at the base and biting off the flesh from inside each leaf. The closer you get to the heart of the artichoke, the more delicate and delicious the flesh becomes. The heart is the choice morsel; to eat it, first remove the flower bristles around it.

Asparagus

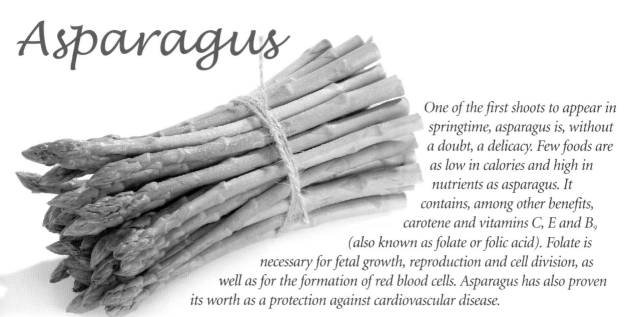

One of the first shoots to appear in springtime, asparagus is, without a doubt, a delicacy. Few foods are as low in calories and high in nutrients as asparagus. It contains, among other benefits, carotene and vitamins C, E and B$_9$ (also known as folate or folic acid). Folate is necessary for fetal growth, reproduction and cell division, as well as for the formation of red blood cells. Asparagus has also proven its worth as a protection against cardiovascular disease.

Health Benefits

- Blood purifier and diuretic
- Lowers cholesterol levels
- Protects against cancer
- Protects against cardiovascular disease
- Replenishes minerals

Put To Good Use

Rich in folate (folic acid), asparagus is particularly recommended for women of childbearing age, especially pregnant women.

Caution

Asparagus is not recommended for people who suffer from gout, rheumatism or cystitis.

Selecting & Storing

Choose asparagus shoots that have rich green, smooth tips that are firm and pointed with a purple tinge. Asparagus can be frozen after being blanched in boiling water. Wrapped in aluminum foil in a hermetically sealed container, it can be kept in the freezer for up to 12 months.

Culinary Use

Served as an appetizer or side dish, asparagus is succulent with a touch of lemon butter or a vinaigrette. It is delicious cold with aioli (see page 223) or in an omelet. To cook, place the shoots in a saucepan, cover with cold water, bring to a boil and simmer for three to five minutes. Eat immediately or rinse with cold water if you plan to eat them later on.

Recipe

- Asparagus in Curry Sauce à l'Orange (page 150)

Healthful Hints

It is preferable to break rather than cut the shoots, but the ends can be peeled to reveal tender flesh. Asparagus is marvelous steamed.

Begin by cooking the largest stalks, then add the smaller ones (which require less cooking time). The stalks can also be cooked in a large casserole pot, standing upright, held together in a bunch with an elastic band, keeping them out of the boiling water to ensure even cooking.

Good To Know

The characteristic "cabbage" odor which may be present in the urine after eating asparagus is caused by a substance called methyl mercaptan. It presents no danger to health.

Avocado

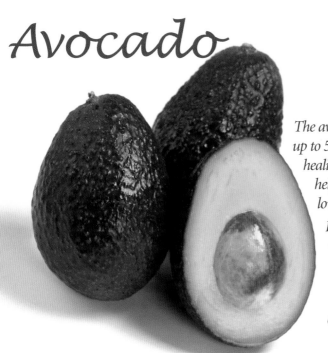

The avocado is a fruit that comes from a tree that grows up to 50 feet (15 m) tall, and it offers incredibly valuable healing properties. It contains monounsaturated fats that help lower blood cholesterol. Do not be put off by its lowly appearance (it was once called the alligator pear) since the flesh of an avocado is fine and luscious. It restores youth and beauty to the skin thanks to its rich vitamin E content. It also contains the antioxidant glutathione that can slow the progress of HIV, as well as folic acid, potassium, and a healthy amount of fiber.

Health Benefits

- Combats HIV
- Lowers hypertension
- Reduces levels of cholesterol
- Relieves constipation
- Slows the aging of cells

Home Remedy

As a purée mixed with lemon juice, avocado works efficiently against constipation.

Caution

The oil in avocados appears to conflict with warfarin, a blood anticoagulant. People who are taking blood thinners should therefore consult their doctor before eating this fruit.

People who are watching their weight should consume avocados in moderation, and avoid adding them to rich foods.

Selecting & Storing

Avocados mature after picking and do not keep for more than a few days at room temperature. The flesh of a mature fruit yields to the touch, this tells you it is ready to eat. To keep slightly longer, store ripe avocados in the refrigerator.

Culinary Use

The fine, delicate flavor of an avocado makes it a delicious appetizer. It is mainly eaten raw since it becomes bitter when cooked. It can be served as an appetizer, puréed in a cold soup, used as a dip (guacamole), a garnish for salmon, crab or shrimp, cut into cubes in salads, or combined with fruits.

To help prevent the darkening of the flesh of an avocado once cut, do not peel or remove the pit of the half to be stored; instead sprinkle the fruit with lemon or lime juice and refrigerate it wrapped in aluminum foil.

Recipes

- Artichoke Apple Avocado Salad (page 216)
- Avocado Dip with Lemon and Anchovy (page 160)
- Pineapple Guacamole (page 149)
- Strawberry Cantaloupe Avocado Salad (page 157)

Healthful Hints

To speed up the ripening of an avocado, store at room temperature in a brown paper bag.

Beauty Secret

Avocado oil softens and smoothes the skin.

Banana

The banana's Latin name, Musa sapientum, *meaning "fruit of the sages," reflects its reputation of having many wonderful health benefits for everyone, from newborns to seniors. It is an excellent source of potassium and vitamin C, and is easy to digest. Rich in calories, the banana is especially highly regarded by athletes because it possesses carbohydrates most efficient for developing muscle mass. Its high concentration of soluble fiber helps to lower cholesterol levels.*

Health Benefits

- Easily digested, highly nutritious
- Effective treatment for diarrhea
- Maintains neurological equilibrium
- Promotes growth of the skeletal system
- Reduces hypertension (high blood pressure)

Home Remedy

People with sensitive stomachs or recurring indigestion are advised to eat a banana every day.

Caution

Unlike plantain, the banana's green Caribbean cousin that must be cooked (see page 98), bananas should be eaten very ripe. Green bananas do not have the same curative and digestive properties.

Because they are rich in carbohydrates, bananas are not recommended for diabetics. For the same reason, they are also not recommended for people trying to lose weight.

Selecting & Storing

Choose bananas that are bright yellow and free of bruises, as these will ripen quickly.

Culinary Use

Eaten raw and combined with cereal grains, bananas make a hearty, flavorful breakfast food. They are a great snack and they add substance to fruit salads. They are especially delicious served with fresh cream.

Recipes

- Bananas with Cinnamon and Rum (page 233)
- Budwig Cream (page 137)
- Fruit Trio Appetizer (page 137)

Healthful Hints

To stop the ripening process of bananas, simply put them in the refrigerator for a few hours. The peels will turn brown but the fruit will remain perfect for eating as long as they are not chilled for too long. On the other hand, to speed up the ripening of green bananas, place them in a paper bag and keep at room temperature.

Fully ripe bananas that cannot be eaten right away can be frozen in sealed plastic bags until needed.

Good To Know

Ink stains on skin can be quickly removed by rubbing with the inner peel of a banana.

B

Barley

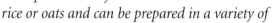

Barley has been consumed by humans since ancient times and it was one of the first cultivated grains. Eaten as a fortifying food, barley has a more pronounced flavor than either rice or oats and can be prepared in a variety of ways. It has numerous health-giving nutrients. In parts of the world where it has been a staple for centuries, notably the Middle East and countries of central Asia, the rate of heart disease is extremely low.

Health Benefits

- Fortifier and diuretic
- Improves digestion
- Inhibits blood coagulation
- Prevents constipation
- Protects again cancer
- Reduces levels of "bad" (LDL) cholesterol

Home Remedy

Drinking or gargling a herbal tea made of barley can relieve a sore throat and calm a cough. Boil 1 oz. (30 g) of hulled barley in 4 cups (1 L) of water for 20 minutes and filter. Drink half a cup at a time, as needed.

Caution

Though barley is integral to the making of beer, do not be mistaken in thinking that the health benefits of barley can be derived from drinking this alcoholic drink. The therapeutic properties of the grain are lost through the various brewing processes.

Selecting & Storing

Among the many different forms in which barley is sold —hulled barley (the grain with its outer husk removed), pearl barley (the de-husked, blanched and mechanically polished grain), barley meal (a coarse-grain flour), barley flakes (rolled, husked grains), and malted barley (sprouted grains used in the food industry)—the best choice, without a doubt, is hulled barley which has a high fiber content and is rich in minerals and thiamin (vitamin B_1).

Culinary Use

The pronounced flavor of barley lends itself best to the preparation of meat stews and hearty winter soups. It can also be a delicious addition to the stuffing for roasted poultry.

Recipes

- Barley Casserole au Gratin (page 194)
- Barley Vege-Paté (page 209)

Healthful Hints

Bearing in mind that barley grains expand to four times their size during cooking, adjust to use a smaller quantity of grain, and be sure to use a large enough cooking pot.

Good To Know

The less barley has been processed, the more its health-giving properties are conserved. It is therefore preferable to consume it as a whole grain (barley-meal flour) or as rolled flakes. Both can be found in health food stores.

Beans, Dried

The white navy bean, the red kidney bean, the speckled pinto bean, the chick-pea (garbanzo), the black bean, the mung bean, the lentil (see page 72) and the soybean (see page 117) are the best known legumes, also called as pulses. Beans are known as the "meat of the poor" since, of all the vegetables, they are the richest in protein. They are also an excellent source of dietary fiber, which protects against cardiovascular disease, and they can have a beneficial preventive effect against certain forms of cancer.

Health Benefits

- Aid and repair nervous system
- Combat obesity
- Help in fetal development
- Help prevent cardiovascular disease
- Help prevent diabetes
- Lower levels of "bad" LDL cholesterol
- Nutritious source of energy
- Reduce the risk of cancer, notably prostate cancer

Put To Good Use

By including cooked dried beans in your diet two or three times a week, you can top up your fiber intake and effectively ward off cardiovascular disease.

Caution

Dried beans commonly cause flatulence if not prepared with care. Soak beans for several hours in water (see below), changing the water several times. Cook in fresh water and discard the water used for soaking.

Selecting & Storing

Dried beans can keep for months in a sealed container. They can also be bought canned since their therapeutic properties are not lost in the canning process.

Culinary Use

Beans and other pulses are found in a multitude of dishes and can be served as dips, vegetable or pasta salads, as vege-paté, or in hearty stews and soups. They can be used to make delicious fried crips, as well as breads, cakes and buns. Before cooking (except in the case of lentils which require no soaking), dried beans must first be softened by soaking in water for four to six hours or overnight. Cook in boiling water after rinsing one last time. Cooking times vary between one and two hours depending on the variety of bean used and how long they have been stored.

B

Recipes

- Chick-Pea Burgers (page 192)
- Chick-Pea Dip (page 160)
- Eggplant Chili (page 197)
- Indian Split Pea Soup (page 174)
- Kidney Bean and Lentil Casserole (page 195)
- Lentil Soup (page 173)
- Lentil Curry with Pistachio (page 193)
- Lentil Terrines with Mushroom (page 155)
- Quiche with Millet, Tofu and Lentils (page 203)
- Tagliatelle with Lentil Sauce (page 208)
- Tofu Chili (page 197)
- Vegetable Chick-Pea Casserole *au Gratin* (page 196)

Great Combinations

All varieties of dried beans go well with finely chopped vegetables such as tomatoes, red or yellow sweet peppers and green onions. The beans are a great source of protein while the vegetables provide vitamins and minerals.

Healthful Hints

How to reduce the soaking time of dried beans

Place beans in water and bring to a boil. Reduce heat and leave to soak in this water, covered, for one hour. Discard water, rinse, then cook according to the cooking time called for in your recipe.

How to lower the incidence of gas caused by beans

Note that the smaller the beans, the easier they are to digest.

Here are a few suggestions to avoid the flatulence (gas) associated with cooked beans:

- If you are not accustomed to eating dried beans, start gradually by eating only a ⅓-cup (75-ml) serving at first.
- Avoid drinking alcohol during the meal.
- Pre-soak the beans several hours before cooking. Change and discard the water used for soaking several times.
- During cooking, add some garlic and ginger, sage, fennel, cumin or savory. Let simmer until well cooked.
- Chew beans well and avoid drinking during the meal.
- Drink plenty of water between meals.
- Avoid eating dessert after a meal containing dried beans.

Good To Know

Canned beans retain all the nutrients of cooked beans and can make a quick meal. They are a highly nutritious substitute for potatoes in soups or as a side dish. They are also an excellent substitute for meat for people wanting to reduce the amount of animal protein in their diet.

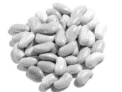
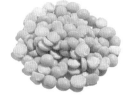

Beans, Fresh

Whether yellow or green, fresh beans all have the same excellent nutrition value. Very low in fat and sodium, and well stocked in potassium, folic acid, fiber and vitamin C, fresh beans are also a source of iron that should not be overlooked.

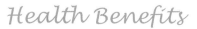

Health Benefits

- Combat infection
- Help in fetal development
- Invigorate
- Stimulate the liver and pancreas

Put To Good Use

Include fresh green or yellow beans in your diet two or three times a week to aid digestion and obtain nutrients essential for good health.

Caution

Avoid overcooking fresh beans so as to take full advantage of their health benefits.

Selecting & Storing

Choose fresh beans with a healthy color, that have not been packaged in cellophane. Discard beans that are stunted, withered, bruised or limp. The more slender the bean, the more tender.

To preserve fresh beans for longer, they can be frozen after blanching for three minutes. These should still be used fairly quickly: within a week or two.

Culinary Use

Cooked fresh beans are an excellent side dish that can add flavor to soups and cold salads. They can be boiled, steamed or prepared in the microwave.

Recipes

- Fresh Beans with Capers and Lemon (page 182)
- Salade Niçoise (page 215)

Great Combinations

Combine green beans with tomatoes (see recipe for Salade Niçoise on page 215) and you have a rich marriage of colors, flavors and nutrients. The carotene and vitamin E in the tomatoes make a great complement to the minerals in the beans, and both are an excellent source of fiber. Drizzled with olive oil and seasoned with minced garlic and parsley, this salad is one of the best preventive "medicines" for your cardiovascular system.

Healthful Hints

Steaming is the best way to ensure that fresh beans retain all their vitamins and nutrients. To avoid overcooking, remove the pot from the stove and uncover as soon as the beans are *al dente* (after about 10 minutes of steaming).

Good To Know

Beans are easy to grow in a garden or in pots on a balcony.

B

Beet

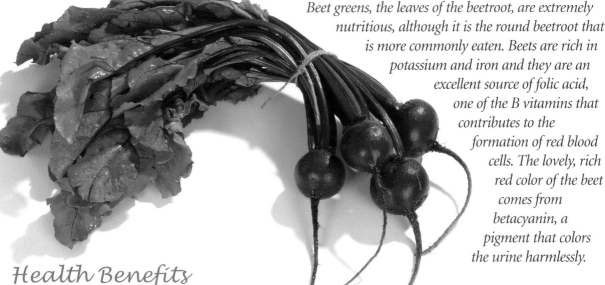

Beet greens, the leaves of the beetroot, are extremely nutritious, although it is the round beetroot that is more commonly eaten. Beets are rich in potassium and iron and they are an excellent source of folic acid, one of the B vitamins that contributes to the formation of red blood cells. The lovely, rich red color of the beet comes from betacyanin, a pigment that colors the urine harmlessly.

Health Benefits

- Aids in the prevention of congenital (fetal) malformation
- Combats anemia
- Excellent source of nutrients and energy
- Highly digestible
- Protects against cardiovascular disease and some forms of cancer
- Relieves constipation

Home Remedy

To fight a cold or anemia, drink a small glass of beet juice every day for a month.

Caution

Beets are not recommended for diabetics.

Selecting & Storing

It is best to choose small- or medium-sized beets since they are easier to cook and peel.

Culinary Use

Raw beet is highly recommended over cooked beet, so as to optimize the vegetable's health and nutrition benefits. If cooking is preferred, it is best to cook with the peel on (to conserve nutrients), either by boiling or by baking in the oven wrapped in aluminum foil.

Recipes

- Beet and Carrot Salad (page 156)
- Buckwheat Muffins with Apple Beet (page 140)

Healthful Hints

Tender beet leaves can be used raw in salads or cooked like spinach, with a little clarified butter.

Good To Know

Canned beets lose very few of their nutrients and health properties, and can thus be consumed all year round with great benefit.

Blueberry

These delicious, small fruits, although not overly rich in nutrients, are an excellent dessert food due to their high fiber content. As with all the other berries, they contain vitamin C, a powerful antioxidant. Vitamin C, it should be noted, is also very important in the prevention of cataracts and eye infections. Blueberries have also been widely used for generations as a cure for diarrhea since they contain a substance that helps to destroy bacteria—particularly E. coli—that cause diarrhea (or other intestinal infections) through poor drinking water or unsanitary conditions.

Health Benefits

- Aids in the prevention of cancer and degenerative diseases
- Astringent, antiseptic, anti-putrefactive
- Combats diabetes
- Helps treat diarrhea
- Improves vision
- Protects the lining of blood vessels
- Relieves venous insufficiency
- Treats inflammations in the mouth

Home Remedy

A handful of fresh blueberries added to your morning cereal enhances the power of your immune system, helping you to efficiently combat colds and infections.

Caution

Blueberries lose their curative properties when cooked. It is therefore better to eat them raw—not a difficult task for most of us!

Selecting & Storing

Choose fruits that are firm with an attractive matte blue color. Refrigerate without washing or covering and consume as soon as possible. They can be frozen once washed and dried, for use in recipes.

Culinary Use

Whether eaten as a snack, with breakfast or for dessert, blueberries are always tasty. Fresh blueberries should be rinsed just before serving, ideally using water to which a spoonful of vinegar has been added.

Recipes

- Blueberry Squares (page 233)
- Blueberry Vinaigrette (page 227)

Beauty Secret

A compress of blueberry water will calm irritated eyes.

Good To Know

Keep in mind the possible presence of pesticide residues on berries and small fruits. Try to opt for organically grown blueberries whenever possible.

B

Broccoli

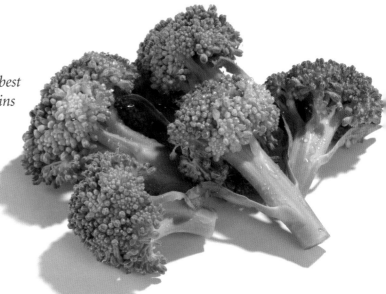

Of all vegetables, broccoli is one of the best sources of vitamin C, and it also contains betas carotene, bringing together two powerful antioxidants. At the same time, broccoli is an important source of dietary fiber. A large number of studies conducted in the U.S. have shown that people who regularly eat broccoli have a reduced risk of developing cancer and cardiovascular disease.

Health Benefits

- Aids in efficient intestinal function
- Invigorates the immune system
- Protects against cardiovascular disease
- Reduces the risk of cancer

Home Remedy

A raw floret of broccoli eaten every day is an efficient protection against infections. It will also diminish the risk of developing cancer.

Caution

We know of no negative properties or contra-indications associated with this excellent healing food. Since the sulfurous flavor of broccoli may be transmitted to breastmilk, some nursing mothers have noticed their baby's dislike for this flavor.

Selecting & Storing

The stems of broccoli should be firm and dark green, the dark green florets small and compact with a hue of violet. Avoid stems that are limp with florets that are yellowing, since these are not fresh. Wrapped in a perforated plastic bag, stems will keep for about a week in the refrigerator.

Culinary Use

Cooked in a broth with zucchini and onions, broccoli makes an excellent addition to a delicious soup. Steamed or cooked in a pressure cooker, it is a great side dish for grilled foods and fish, or it can be a savory appetizer *au gratin*. Raw broccoli gives a satisfying crunch to salads and can contribute to a healthy, eye-catching arrangement of crudités (raw vegetables) with dip.

Recipe

- Broccoli Soup (page 167)

Healthful Hints

To preserve broccoli longer, simply separate florets into similar-sized bunches, blanch and freeze. Will keep frozen for up to six months.

Good To Know

Broccoli loses a few nutrients in cooking, and microwave cooking causes it to lose even more of its benefits. The rule of thumb, therefore, is to eat the vegetable raw wherever possible.

Buckwheat

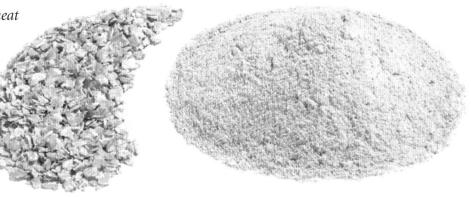

The seeds of the buckwheat plant, from the same family as rhubarb and sorrel, are a "complete food" that contain amine compounds. These have a reputation for inhibiting the development of cancer. Buckwheat, also known by some as kasha, is rich in rutin, a flavonoid and antioxidant that improves blood circulation and reduces hypertension. Because buckwheat does not contain gluten, it is strongly recommended for people with celiac disease or those suffering from digestive problems.

Health Benefits

- Aids in the prevention of hemorrhaging
- Improves blood circulation
- Reduces high blood pressure
- Relieves digestive problems

Put To Good Use

Buckwheat is highly recommended for diabetics because the carbohydrates it contains are very slowly digested. Owing to its hunger-satisfying properties, it is also prescribed to people who are trying to lose weight.

Caution

Contrary to common sense, low-calorie buckwheat flour is recommended by specialists over wholegrain buckwheat flour because it contains more nutrients.

Selecting & Storing

Buckwheat can be stored just like other flours: in a sealed container away from humidity and direct light.

Culinary Use

Buckwheat flour is used most commonly to make pancakes and cakes, while the whole grain (kasha) can be made into a hearty porridge or delicious puddings.

Recipes

- Buckwheat Muffins with Apple and Beet (page 140)
- Buckwheat Pancakes (page 138)
- Buckwheat Vege-Pâté (page 159)
- Budwig Cream (page 137)
- Zucchini Buckwheat Loaf Cake (page 238)
- Zucchini Chocolate Loaf Cake (page 237)

Healthful Hints

Wheat flour can be replaced by buckwheat flour in many cake, muffin and crisp recipes.

Good To Know

Buckwheat is widely eaten in Japan: another likely factor to explain the nation's low incidence of cancer and cardiovascular disease.

B

Cabbage

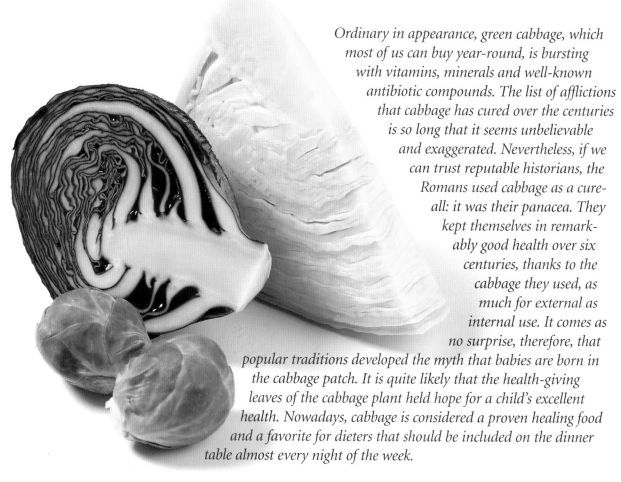

Ordinary in appearance, green cabbage, which most of us can buy year-round, is bursting with vitamins, minerals and well-known antibiotic compounds. The list of afflictions that cabbage has cured over the centuries is so long that it seems unbelievable and exaggerated. Nevertheless, if we can trust reputable historians, the Romans used cabbage as a cure-all: it was their panacea. They kept themselves in remarkably good health over six centuries, thanks to the cabbage they used, as much for external as internal use. It comes as no surprise, therefore, that popular traditions developed the myth that babies are born in the cabbage patch. It is quite likely that the health-giving leaves of the cabbage plant held hope for a child's excellent health. Nowadays, cabbage is considered a proven healing food and a favorite for dieters that should be included on the dinner table almost every night of the week.

Health Benefits

- Aids in growth
- Helps destroy viruses
- Helps heal external wounds
- Helps heal ulcers and hernias
- Protects against colds
- Reduces the risk of cancer, notably of the stomach and colon
- Relieves arthritis, rheumatism and shingles

Put To Good Use

Eating raw cabbage at least three times a week is, without question, a highly effective protection against a variety of afflictions, including cancer.

Caution

Raw or steamed, cabbage can be eaten by everyone. However, in order to retain all the healing nutrients, avoid cooking it immersed in water.

Selecting & Storing

Choose a head of green cabbage that is heavy, with leaves that are green and firm, without marks, spots or tears. This hearty vegetable will keep for a month in the refrigerator in a plastic bag. Savoy cabbage has curly, crinkled dark green leaves that keep their form once cooked. Bok choy (pak choi or Chinese cabbage) is the darling of Asian chefs.

It has large, deep green leaves and long, pure white stems that resemble celery stalks.

Culinary Use

Forget about soggy, bland, humdrum cabbage salads, and prepare to discover new qualities in raw cabbage. Sliced into strips, mixed into fresh salad and drizzled with a simple vinaigrette made with olive oil and lemon juice, cabbage possesses a whole new flavor. Mix with your favorite vegetables and fruits (such as apples, pears or clementines) and you have a refreshing appetizer that really awakens the senses. Choose a very young cabbage and remove its tough outer leaves and fibrous core before preparing. It is best served as an appetizer, sprinkled with dressing, with diced apples, an assortment of lettuce leaves and almonds (see recipes below). Steamed or stir-fried, the leaves of bok choy taste like spinach, while the stalks taste like celery.

Recipes

- Cabbage Salad with Clementine, Spinach and Sesame (page 215)
- Chinese Cabbage Rolls (page 205)
- Artichoke Apple Avocado Salad (page 216)
- Sautéed Brussels Sprouts (page 180)

Great Combinations

Pair up cabbage and shredded carrots and you will discover a powerful combination of antioxidants.

Healthful Hints

Cabbage salad is more delicious if strips of the vegetable are allowed to soak in water for 30 minutes before preparing. The salad is also better if refrigerated for 30 minutes before eating.

Beauty Secret

The cabbage mask

Experts recommend applying cabbage leaves to the face for half an hour (much like applying a beauty mask) to absorb toxins and impurities and to regenerate the skin tissues.

Other Varieties

Savoy cabbage is similar to regular green cabbage, except for its textured, rich green leaves. Napa, also called Chinese cabbage, has a more delicate flavor. Bok choy, another Chinese green vegetable, is a variety that is usually served cooked. Red cabbage, white cabbage (pale green in color) and Brussels sprouts all possess healing properties similar to green cabbage.

Good To Know

Some advice to fans of sauerkraut: this pickled and fermented cabbage food is very good for you as long as it is prepared traditionally and not processed industrially. As a pickled food, it is not recommended for people on a low-sodium diet. What is likely indigestible about sauerkraut are all the rich meats that tend to be eaten in excess alongside it.

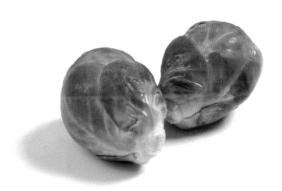

C

Cantaloupe

In addition to being a succulent fruit, the cantaloupe melon is bursting with beneficial properties. Among the many varieties of melon found around the world, the cantaloupe, a variety of muskmelon, is one of the most popular. It is also one of the most nutritious melons by virtue of its levels of vitamin C, beta carotene, minerals and folate (folic acid).

Selecting & Storing

Choose a melon that is heavy, without bruises or blemishes. Since a cantaloupe does not mature further once picked, be sure to choose one that is ripe and has a slight depression where its stem was attached. A ripe melon should have a pleasant odor. This odor is very pronounced in overripe fruit on the verge of spoiling. Avoid melons without aroma or those with a strong odor. Ripe cantaloupe must be eaten within a day or so and will not keep.

Health Benefits

- Aids in the prevention of cataracts
- Anticoagulant and combats anemia
- Diuretic and laxative
- Lowers blood pressure
- Rejuvenates tissues
- Reduces the risk of cancer
- Relieves rheumatism and gout
- Stimulates appetite

Home Remedy

People suffering from high blood pressure have noticed a marked improvement in their condition simply by eating a slice of cantaloupe before each meal. These same people have also benefited from the fruit's cancer-fighting properties.

Caution

Cantaloupe is not recommended for diabetics or people suffering intestinal enteritis or indigestion (dyspepsia). People with Oral Allergy Syndrome (see page 86) may experience a reaction.

Culinary Use

The Italians are wise to serve fresh melon as an appetizer, for this is the best way to elicit the fruit's healing properties. Add chunks of cantaloupe to lettuce and cabbage salads; its color and sweet flavor will make them irresistible.

Recipes

- Cantaloupe with Chèvre and Porto (page 151)
- Strawberry Cantaloupe Avocado Salad (page 157)

Beauty Secret

Applied daily to the face, a mixture of equal parts melon juice, milk and distilled water works to combat dry skin.

Good To Know

As with most fruits, it is preferable to eat cantaloupe before a meal. A little salt and pepper makes the melon easier to digest.

Carrot

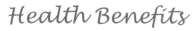

As we all know, carrots are an excellent source of beta carotene, as well as potassium and fiber. The health benefits are just too numerous to count; carrots are one of the healing foods with the greatest number of therapeutic properties. The reinvigorating juice of carrots is highly beneficial to the liver.

Health Benefits

- Bolsters the immune system
- Combats anemia
- Combats bacterial infections
- Improves night vision
- Reduces blood cholesterol
- Relieves both constipation and diarrhea
- Restores minerals and invigorates

Put To Good Use

Eating a raw carrot every day is tantamount to taking a natural medicine that is bursting with health-giving properties. It has been proven that people who consume carrots every day are less likely to develop macular degeneration (reduction of central vision) and cardiovascular disease.

Caution

To enjoy all the healing properties of carrots, it is preferable not to peel them. Choose organically grown carrots that have not been treated, and simply scrape or brush away any dirt while washing.

Selecting & Storing

Carrots sold with their leaves intact generally have a better flavor. All carrots will keep for several weeks in the refrigerator.

Culinary Use

Carrots can be cooked in a variety of ways. They are excellent in soups, as appetizers and side dishes, and can be included in the baking of delicious cakes, cookies and muffins. The juice of carrots is exquisite and full of healthy nutrients. Their leaves, too, can be added to soups, as well as salads and sauces.

Recipes

- Beet and Carrot Salad (page 156)
- Carrots and Parsnips with Dulse (page 151)
- Mashed Potatoes with Carrot and Rutabaga (page 184)

Healthful Hints

Add 1 tbsp (15 ml) of lemon juice to the cooking water to improve the flavor of soft carrots. Though the lemon will lighten the color of the carrots slightly, it will stop them from discoloring.

Beauty Secret

Carrot juice, applied as a lotion to the face and neck, softens the skin and will protect against wrinkles.

Good To Know

Carrots do not lose their health-giving properties through cooking. People who eat a great many carrots might develop yellowish skin, but this is not dangerous and will quickly disappear once a regular diet is resumed.

C

Cauliflower

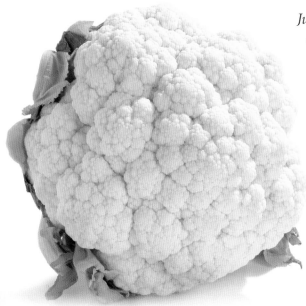

Just like its other relatives in the cabbage-mustard family, cauliflower is a vegetable that protects against several forms of cancer. Low in calories, fat and sodium, it is an excellent source of dietary fiber, minerals such as phosphorus, iron and potassium, and vitamin C.

Health Benefits

- Inhibits the growth of tumors
- Protects against breast, colon and prostate cancer
- Protects against colds and the flu
- Stimulates the immune system

Put To Good Use

A 3-oz. (100-g) serving of raw cauliflower every day supplies the daily amount of vitamin C recommended by nutritionists.

Caution

Cauliflower can cause flatulence as the intestines digest the cellulose it contains.

People suffering from gout should avoid this vegetable, choosing instead cabbage or broccoli which contain fewer amino acids. The puric acid found in cauliflower can cause painful episodes of gout.

Selecting & Storing

Choose a head of cauliflower that is heavy, with rich green leaves and florets that are a creamy-white color. Brown marks on the florets are an indication that the cauliflower is not fresh. If it cannot be eaten the same day, avoid washing the cauliflower and refrigerate—but always wash before use. Stored in a perforated plastic bag, it will keep for about a week.

Culinary Use

Cooked in a broth by itself, or with carrots or broccoli, cauliflower makes for savory soups with a lovely texture. Used raw, its white florets have a pleasing crunch that adds variety to a green salad or a platter of crudités. Cauliflower is also excellent for satisfying the appetite.

Recipes

- Cauliflower Soup (page 168)
- Indian-Style Braised Cauliflower (page 179)

Healthful Hints

In cooked dishes of cauliflower, the yellowing of the florets can be prevented by adding lemon juice to the boiling water.

The sulfurous odor that is released during cooking will be less concentrated in cauliflower if it is boiled uncovered in water to which a whole, unshelled walnut has been added.

Good To Know

Cauliflower is the most easily digested vegetable in the cabbage family.

Celeriac

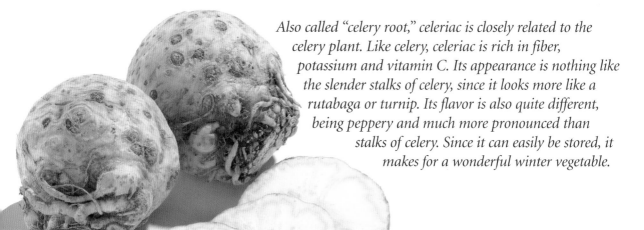

Also called "celery root," celeriac is closely related to the celery plant. Like celery, celeriac is rich in fiber, potassium and vitamin C. Its appearance is nothing like the slender stalks of celery, since it looks more like a rutabaga or turnip. Its flavor is also quite different, being peppery and much more pronounced than stalks of celery. Since it can easily be stored, it makes for a wonderful winter vegetable.

Culinary Use

Not commonly used in North America, celeriac is widely appreciated in Europe where it is often served raw on platters of crudités. Cooked, it is used in tasty soups, mashed or baked *au gratin*. Raw, it is used in salads or served on its own, sprinkled with vinaigrette.

Health Benefits

- Aids and invigorates digestion
- Anti-rheumatic
- Antiseptic
- Stimulates appetite, freshens the palate
- Stimulates the adrenal glands

Recipe

- Sweet Potato and Celeriac Soup (page 171)

Great Combinations

Combine celeriac, carrots and Gruyere cheese to make a purée that needs no salt, since celeriac is already rich in sodium. This vitamin-rich purée is also enhanced with protein and calcium (supplied by the Gruyere).

Home Remedy

Served raw in a salad and eaten twice a week, this root vegetable improves digestion.

Caution

As with celery stalks, celeriac is rich in sodium and is therefore not recommended for people on a low-sodium diet.

Healthful Hints

Because the flesh of this root rapidly darkens in color when exposed to air, it should be brushed with lemon juice or immersed in salt water with some lemon juice added.

Selecting & Storing

Choose a celeriac root that is free of bruises and blemishes. This vegetable will keep for over a week in the refrigerator.

Good To Know

Of all vegetables, celeriac contains the highest levels of sodium.

C

Celery

This vegetable, while rich in dietary fiber, is about 95 percent water. The vitamins A and C it contains are found mainly in its leaves, along with most of its calcium, iron and potassium. According to recent studies, its high content of complex nutrients may play a part in inhibiting the growth of tumor cells. Celery juice applied directly on a wound promotes speedy healing. Low in calories, it is recommended as a hunger suppressant for people wanting to lose weight.

Health Benefits

- Aids in protecting against cancer
- Astringent that aids digestion
- Lowers blood pressure
- Relieves rheumatism

Home Remedies

Hypertension (high blood pressure)

For people with hypertension, it is advisable to eat four or five stalks of celery every day for a week, then stop for three weeks before beginning to consume celery on a daily basis once more.

Rheumatism

A half-glass of celery juice every day for 15 days is recommended for people suffering from rheumatism.

Caution

Since the leaves and seeds of celery are rich in sodium, they are not recommended for people on a low-sodium diet.

Selecting & Storing

Be sure to choose celery with branches and leaves that are firm and fresh and are a pleasing green color. In the refrigerator, it can be kept for over a week in a perforated plastic bag. To restore vigor and crunch to wilted celery, place in cold water and refrigerate for a few hours.

Culinary Use

Celery is generally eaten raw but it also adds a lovely flavor to soups, sauces and stews.

Recipe

- Curried Celery Soup (page 171)

Healthful Hints

A stalk of celery cut into small sticks (julienne-style) can be added to sauces and stews 15 minutes before the end of cooking to give a pleasing crunch to their texture.

Good To Know

Celery does not lose its nutrients with cooking. However, it will lose nutrients when soaked in water or liquid.

Cherry

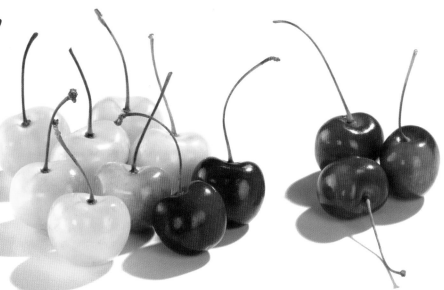

Despite being rich in sugar, cherries are recommended for diabetics since the sugar is in a form called fructose, which is more slowly assimilated by the blood. This delicious fruit is also considered to be a hunger suppressant and is packed with vitamins and minerals. Traditional and popular medicine contend that cherries heal gout and rheumatism. While some research has denied this, several other studies have recognized definite therapeutic properties that may relieve these medical conditions.

Health Benefits

- Anti-rheumatic and anti-arthritic
- Detoxifies and purifies tissues
- Diuretic
- Improves intestinal function
- Reduces the risk of cardiovascular disease
- Regulates the liver and stomach
- Relieves gout

Home Remedy

Cleaning house

An excellent way to eliminate waste and stored toxins in the body is to eat a diet of only cherries for one or two days.

Recipe to alleviate gout

Place a handful of cherry stems in a saucepan with 4 cups (1 liter) of boiling water, lower the heat and leave to simmer for 7 to 10 minutes. Remove from the heat and allow to cool, covered, for 20 minutes. Drink 2 cups (500 ml) per day.

Caution

Avoid drinking water after eating cherries since it will cause the cellulose in the stomach to bloat.

Raw cherries are not recommended for people suffering from indigestion or for those with a sensitive stomach. Instead, cherries can be eaten cooked as a fruit sauce, or in jams or jellies. People with Oral Allergy Syndrome (see entry for Orange on page 86) may experience itching in the mouth and anaphylaxis from eating cherries and should thus avoid the fruit.

People wishing to lose weight should avoid cherries, not only because they are high in calories, but because they are so easy to snack on—and to overeat!

Culinary Use

Cherries can be cooked into delicious jams, preserves and pies, but very few of their health benefits are retained this way; it is much better to eat them raw. They can also be made into a delicious juice.

C

Selecting & Storing

Sugary-sweet Bing cherries are firm and smooth with a lovely, dark red color. Morello (or sour) cherries, with their acidic flesh, are a yellow-red color or clear, bright red. The stems should always be green since black stems are an indication that the fruit is not fresh. Avoid washing cherries before refrigerating, but always wash before eating.

Recipes

- Fruit Trio Appetizer (page 137)
- Orange and Cherry Soy Smoothie (page 135)

Healthful Hints

For cherries to be enjoyed throughout the year, they can be frozen, as long as care is taken to remove the pits. As with strawberries, spread them in a single layer on a cookie sheet and place in the freezer for several hours. Then put into sealed containers to keep for up to six months. Dried cherries will keep for about a year in a sealed container.

Great Combinations

A salad of red fruits (such as cherries, strawberries and raspberries) is a refreshing and invigorating snack, chock-full of vitamins. It is also a potent cell fortifier thanks to the antioxidants of these small fruits. Such a salad also helps to improve intestinal regularity and enhances kidney function.

Beauty Secret

Crushed cherries are an excellent invigorator for the skin of the face and neck.

Good To Know

Maraschino cherries are bathed in sugary syrup, food coloring and chemical preservatives, and therefore contain negligible nutritional value.

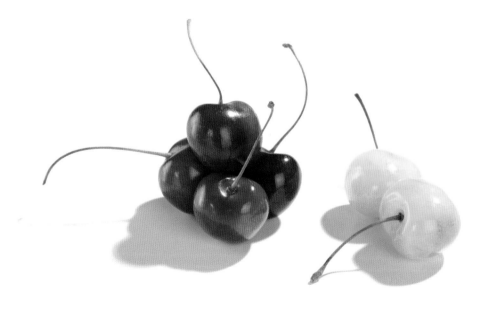

Cinnamon

If it can be said that music soothes the soul, then cinnamon, one of the oldest known spices, combats the foul humors of even the most unpleasant grouches. The spice contains eugenol, a natural analgesic that gives a sense of well-being. Cinnamon is also a good source of iron and calcium. Traditionally, it has been used as a remedy to relieve stomach pain and intestinal gas. It has also been found to help the body increase the production of insulin. Recent studies have shown that the spice helps the intestines to function.

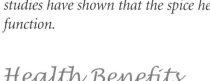

Health Benefits

- Anti-bacterial
- Combats flatulence
- Improves intestinal function
- Increases the body's production of insulin
- Relieves stomach pain
- Soothes pain

Put To Good Use

You only need a little cinnamon to benefit from its ability to increase insulin levels or improve digestion. Sprinkling a little cinnamon on your morning toast adds a little burst of good cheer to the day.

Caution

The essential oil of cinnamon that is used in aromatherapy for its stimulating odor, is said to activate both the libido and the mind. This oil, however, should never be taken internally or used as a seasoning.

Selecting & Storing

Cinnamon is sold either in quills (sticks) of curled bark or in powdered form. Like all spices, it is best preserved in a dry place out of the light.

Culinary Use

This spice is not only excellent for lending a delicious aroma to desserts; it also lends its unique flavor to hot beverages such as herbal tea and hot cider. Some Asian and African cultures use it in their cooking to add a fuller flavor to meat dishes.

Recipes

- Bananas with Cinnamon and Rum (page 233)
- Beet and Carrot Salad (page 156)
- Hot Cider with Cinnamon (page 245)

Healthful Hints

To make a cinnamon herb tea, drop a few pieces of cinnamon stick into a cup of boiling water and steep for 10 minutes.

Good To Know

Cinnamon is an inexpensive antiseptic that works efficiently to treat infections. Apply a pinch or two of cinnamon to scrapes or shallow cuts to relieve pain quickly.

C

Clementine

This relative of the mandarin orange is a similar small fruit that is now available to us several months of the year. The clementine is a favorite with children, who adore its sweetness and easy-to-remove peel. In addition to being a rich source of vitamin C, it contains flavonoids (also called vitamin P) that enhance the antioxidant action of vitamin C.

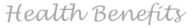

Health Benefits

- Helps in the prevention of colds
- Reduces the risk of developing cancer
- Stimulates the appetite and digestion

Put To Good Use

Eating two clementines a day will give you half the recommended daily amount of vitamin C.

Caution

This fruit can generally be eaten and enjoyed by everyone, although some people may experience itching in the mouth from eating clementines due to Oral Allergy Syndrome (see entry for Orange on page 86). In this case, the fruit should be avoided.

Selecting & Storing

It is best to choose fruit that seem heavy for their size since these are the juiciest. They generally keep for well over a week at room temperature or in the refrigerator.

Culinary Use

Clementines are usually eaten as a snack but they are equally delicious in fruit salads. Wedges of clementine can also be added to leafy vegetable salads or pasta salads.

Recipes

- Apricot, Fig and Clementine Purée (page 135)
- Cabbage Salad with Spinach, Clementine and Sesame (page 215)

Great Combinations

Try combining clementine, yogurt, honey and a touch of lemon juice. The calcium from the yogurt is readily absorbed thanks to the presence of organic acids and vitamin C in the citrus juice.

Healthful Hints

Because it is so easy to peel, the clementine is a great replacement for oranges if you are in a rush to prepare a salad.

Good To Know

Along with the tangerine and mandarin, new varieties of citrus fruits like the clementine are the result of crossing different hybrids. The ugli fruit from Jamaica looks like a deformed grapefruit. Its pulp is juicier and a bit more acidic than the pomelo, a Southeast Asian grapefruit. The tangelo is a cross between the mandarin orange and the grapefruit. It is juicier and less acidic than the pomelo.

Cocoa and Chocolate

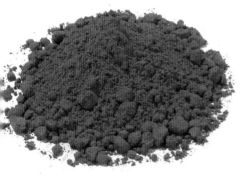

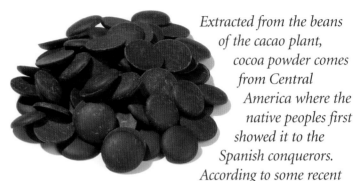

Extracted from the beans of the cacao plant, cocoa powder comes from Central America where the native peoples first showed it to the Spanish conquerors. According to some recent studies conducted in the U.S., pure cocoa is twice as rich in a certain type of polyphenol antioxidant as a glass of red wine, and three times richer than a cup of green tea. Cocoa is also an excellent source of copper, potassium, vitamin B_{12} and iron. It contains tannins and flavonoids, as well as a significant quantity of dietary fiber. The only way to benefit from the medicinal properties of cocoa and chocolate is to eat high-quality dark chocolate (bittersweet or semi-sweet chocolate, which contain over 70 percent cocoa and cocoa butter, along with lecithin and vanilla).

Health Benefits

- Combats high blood pressure (hypertension)
- Energizes
- Has a positive effect on blood coagulation
- Improves the elasticity of the blood vessels
- Increases the levels of "good" (HDL) cholesterol
- Protects again cardiovascular disease
- Stimulates the digestive system

Put To Good Use

A cup of hot chocolate works to combat the aging of cells and protects against heart disease and cancer. However, be careful not to use cow's milk (see the Not-So-Great Combination below); instead, prepare it as a rice- or soy-based drink.

As an effective prevention against cancer, many oncologists who uphold the healing powers of foods recommend that we eat about three-quarters of an ounce (20 grams) of dark chocolate daily.

Caution

Yes, cocoa powder and chocolate are good for one's health...but watch the sugar content and calories. Avoid chocolate candies and milk chocolate; instead, select pure dark chocolate. Moderation should be the rule of thumb: only a modest amount of chocolate should be consumed.

Cocoa and chocolate contain stimulants, notably theobromine and caffeine; another good reason to exercise moderation in your consumption of these foods.

Chocolate is not recommended for people who suffer from migraines or acid reflux.

Selecting & Storing

Chocolate obtained from a specialty shops will generally be of better quality than products bought in a supermarket or grocery store. Carefully check the ingredient labels for the

C

percentage of cocoa content. The higher the percentage of cocoa, the greater the healing benefits. High-quality chocolate is smooth and snaps cleanly when broken. Avoid products with a lumpy texture, those that are covered with whitish powder, or those that crumble instead of breaking. Dark chocolate keeps for about a month when stored in a cool place. Cocoa powder will keep for up to six months in a cool, dry place.

Culinary Use

Cocoa powder is used in baking and pastry making and is the basic ingredient of chocolate. Certain cultures combine it with poultry and lamb: a well-known Mexican dish called *mole poblano* combines cocoa with turkey or chicken.

Recipes

- Dairy-Free Chocolate Icing (page 237)
- Zucchini Chocolate Loaf Cake (page 237)

A Not-So-Great Combination

It should be noted that an unfortunate conflict occurs in the popular combination of cow's milk and cocoa. As demonstrated in a recent study, the proteins in milk counteract the flavonoids of cocoa (its principal medicinal component). For this reason, dark chocolate is much better for you than milk chocolate or hot chocolate made with milk.

Healthful Hints

Cocoa powder is not easily mixed into a liquid and tends to clump together. To avoid this, first mix together the cocoa and sugar, then add a little cold liquid a few drops at a time, mixing it into a paste before adding to a soy or rice drink.

Remedy for mothers

Cocoa butter contains a soothing property that helps to prevent the cracked nipples of women who are breastfeeding.

Good To Know

Chocolate contains saturated fats, but these are fats that are not a danger to the system. On the contrary, they appear to exercise a positive effect on the cardiovascular system. The greater the percentage of cocoa in chocolate, the less sugar it usually contains. The flavor is therefore both more pronounced and more bitter.

White chocolate does not contain the flavonoids of dark chocolate since it is made only from cocoa butter.

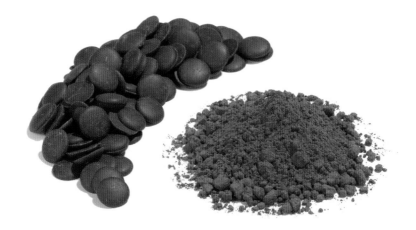

Coconut

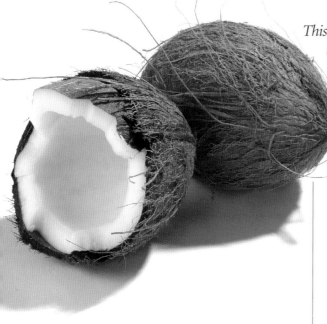

This large fruit of the coconut palm tree is lower in minerals and vitamin E than other nuts. On the other hand, it is especially rich in dietary fiber, making it an excellent healing food. Since it contains a high concentration of saturated fats which inhibit its decomposition, coconut oil is commonly used in the food industry.

Health Benefits

- Aids in the absorption of dietary fats
- Diuretic and laxative
- Protects against cardiovascular disease

Put To Good Use

To take best advantage of the medicinal benefits of coconut, it is best to use unsweetened flakes.

Caution

Richer in saturated fats than the most calorie-rich meats or nuts, coconut should be consumed in moderation.

Selecting & Storing

Dried, shredded coconut—the most popular form of the nut—can be obtained almost anywhere. When buying a fresh, whole coconut, choose one that still has its water. (Coconut water is not the same as coconut milk, which is a richer mixture. See recipe below and on page 247.) To check for coconut water, simply listen carefully as you shake the nut. Dried coconut can be kept at room temperature for one or two months. Keep fresh coconut and coconut milk in the refrigerator.

Culinary Use

Shredded coconut gives flavor and texture to a variety of desserts, while prepared coconut milk (see page 247)—made from a rich mixture of coconut—is used to perfume curry, rice and seafood dishes.

Recipes

- Coconut Milk (page 247)
- Crème Caramel with Coconut Milk (page 235)
- Homemade Granola (page 139)

Healthful Hints

The very best way to open a coconut is as follows: first, pierce one of the three "eyes" of the coconut and drain the water. Place the nut in an oven heated to 350°F (180°C) and heat for 15 minutes. Once removed from the oven, a swift blow with a hammer should easily open the nut.

Good To Know

How to make coconut milk

Blend 1 cup (250 ml) of grated coconut with 2 cups (500 ml) of boiling water. Once mixed, let the liquid cool before filtering it through a cheesecloth. Let stand until the coconut milk layer rises to the top, like cream separating from milk. Coconut milk will keep for only one or two days in the refrigerator, but it can be frozen.

C

Corn

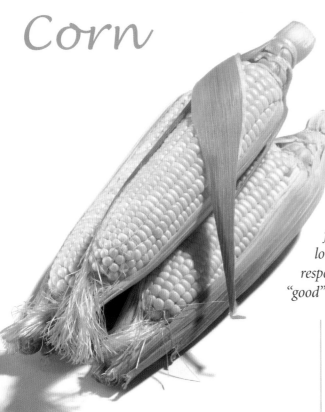

A summertime favorite, sweet, crunchy corn on the cob is actually a cereal grain that has been harvested before reaching maturity. Rich in dietary fiber, fresh corn aids in lowering levels of "bad" (LDL) cholesterol in the system. The carbohydrate content in corn provides a quick supply of energy to the body without the usual fats. Corn oil, which has now been shown to also lower the "bad" (LDL) cholesterol in the blood, is also responsible—unfortunately—for reducing levels of "good" cholesterol (known as HDL).

Health Benefits

- Nutritious and a good source of energy
- Protects against dental cavities
- Reduces the risk of cancer
- Restores tone in muscles and other tissues

Put To Good Use

Consumed in moderation once or twice a week, steamed corn supplies an abundance of energy and an appreciable amount of vitamin E.

Caution

Many people who suffer from Irritable Bowel Syndrome (IBS) have noticed an increase in painful symptoms after eating corn. If this is your situation, be wary of the corn found in the foods you eat, particularly in breakfast cereals. Industrially processed foods and ingredients derived from corn are responsible for a number of allergies.

Selecting & Storing

Choose cobs of corn that are fully ripe, where the kernels are large and juicy, the juice being milky in color. White corn is preferred to yellow corn since it contains twice as much dietary fiber. Since corn loses a number of its beneficial properties during storage, it is always best to eat it as fresh as possible.

Culinary Use

Even though we may be in the habit of boiling corn in water, or a mixture of milk and water, it is preferable to steam corn to maximize the full range of its health benefits and healing properties.

Recipe

- Corn and Quinoa Soup (page 174)

Healthful Hints

Corn on the cob cooked for a few minutes in the pressure cooker, or even grilled on the barbecue, is a real delicacy.

Good To Know

Popcorn is good for your health as long as it isn't drenched in melted butter or doused in salt.

Cranberry

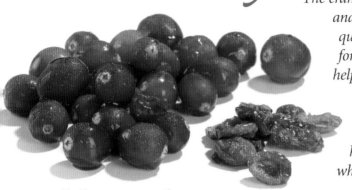

The cranberry is an excellent source of dietary fiber and vitamin C and has a high concentration of quinic acid, which makes it an effective remedy for treating bladder infections (cystitis) and helping in the prevention of kidney stones and gallstones. It also contains an antibiotic compound that, as in blueberries, fortifies the linings and membranes of organs to help prevent bacterial infections, some of which have been linked to cancer.

Health Benefits

- Antibiotic and bactericide
- Helps improve vision and protects against eye infection
- Helps prevent urinary tract infections

Put To Good Use

Two small glasses (1 ½ cups/375 ml) of cranberry juice a day offer a good protection against urinary tract infections.

Caution

Bottled cranberry juice tends to contain excess sugar and other sweeteners. It is preferable to make your own cranberry juice with a juice extractor whenever possible.

Despite the documented antibiotic effects of cranberry, the juice of this fruit should not be taken as a replacement for antibiotics prescribed by a physician for a urinary tract infection.

Diabetics must be careful to take only sugar-free cranberry tablets or drink pure, unsweetened juice, since cranberry "cocktails" and drinks may contain glucose as well as fructose.

Selecting & Storing

Choose plump, firm, shiny fruit with an appealing red color. Do not wash fresh cranberries until ready to use. They keep well in the refrigerator, for up to two months. Naturally sweetened dried cranberries are a convenient form of this fruit.

Culinary Use

Due to the slightly sour, acidic flavor of raw cranberries, cooked cranberries are preferable. They are used in cakes, cookies and muffins. As they cook, they need only a very little water. It is advised to cover them while cooking since they will swell and burst as they start to boil. Cranberries are delicious in chutneys, jams, fruit sauces and jellies.

Recipes

- Cranberry Sauce with Orange and Ginger (page 225)
- Cranberry-Strawberry Purée (page 234)

Healthful Hints

To use less of sugar needed for cooking cranberries, replace some of the water with apple juice.

Beauty Secret

Cranberries are used more and more in making cosmetics and beauty products. Mix a small amount of cranberry juice with make-up remover and apply to the face and neck to liven the complexion.

Good To Know

Recent studies conducted in Canada have shown that cranberry extract may be effective against some intestinal viruses.

C

Cress

Renowned since ancient times for its medicinal properties, cress is a fortifying green vegetable with the reputation of curing scurvy: it contains almost as much vitamin C as lemon. Also available in other varieties (land cress, curly cress and watercress), it is rich in vitamins A and B, and is a good source of iron, iodine, phosphorus, calcium, sodium and potassium.

Health Benefits

- Antidote for nicotine
- Combats anemia
- Detoxifies the system
- Diuretic
- Protects against cardiovascular disease
- Stimulates appetite

Put To Good Use

Try blending or even replacing lettuce with cress in sandwiches and salads as an effective protection against a variety of ailments.

Smokers should make an effort to eat cress on a daily basis since it has been found that this leafy vegetable offers protection against lung cancer through its neutralizing effect on nicotine.

Caution

Too much cress may cause an upset stomach for some people; it may also cause urinary tract problems.

Selecting & Storing

Choose a bunch of cress with leaves that are undamaged and a healthy green color. Store in a plastic bag in the refrigerator. Cress can also be placed in a glass jar with a little water and sealed with plastic wrap to keep the leaves fresh and crisp. Cress should be eaten as soon as possible and will not keep for longer than four or five days.

Culinary Use

Cress and watercress can be cooked, though this will destroy many of its health-giving properties. Cress is best added raw to salads mixed with lettuce, or used as a garnish for a platter of raw vegetables to create a veritable smorgasbord of vitamins.

Recipe

- Cress Salad with Apple, Hazelnut and Chèvre (page 156)

Beauty Secret

A weekly scalp massage of cress juice will help slow down—or even stop—hair loss.

Good To Know

A 3-oz. (100-g) portion of cress contains more vitamin C than the daily recommended amount.

Eggplant

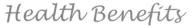

This lovely, pear-shaped vegetable has a rich, deep maroon color. It has few calories and is easily digested. Though low in protein, carbohydrates and fats, it is quite rich in potassium, which contributes to its diuretic property. According to recent research, eggplant has been shown to inhibit the rise of blood lipid and cholesterol levels after a meal rich in fatty foods.

Health Benefits

- Anti-rheumatic
- Combats anemia
- Reduces "bad" (LDL) cholesterol
- Shown to prevent some forms of cancer in laboratory animals
- Stimulates the liver and pancreas

Put To Good Use

It is advisable to eat eggplant once a week to reduce levels of "bad" (LDL) cholesterol.

Caution

Although eggplant itself is low in calories, it readily absorbs fats and oil during cooking. It is therefore preferable to eat the vegetable raw in appetizers and hors d'oeuvres, steamed, or cooked in sauces and stews.

Selecting & Storing

The skin of an eggplant should be firm and smooth to the touch, with an attractive deep purple color, while the stalk should be prickly and healthy green. Eggplants keep for several days in the refrigerator. Their skins will shrivel as they dehydrate. Wrinkled eggplants become slightly bitter and are not as good for eating. Eggplant is ripe when a light touch of the finger leaves an impression on its surface.

Recipes

- Eggplant Chili (page 197)
- Ratatouille Niçoise (page 155)
- Spaghetti with Eggplant and Shiitake Mushrooms (page 207)

Culinary Use

A number of countries use eggplant in a variety of delicious traditional dishes: moussaka (Greece), ratatouille (France), baba ganoush (Lebanon), and aubergine parmigiana (Italy). Eggplant adds a unique flavor to tomato sauce, as you will see in the recipes recommended above.

Healthful Hints

To remove the bitter flavor, cut eggplant into slices, sprinkle with salt and leave to "sweat" for 30 minutes. Then rinse with water and dry with a paper towel.

Good To Know

The younger the eggplant, the more tender and less bitter it will be. Choose eggplants that are longer in shape since they have fewer seeds (which are the source of the bitter taste).

E

Endive

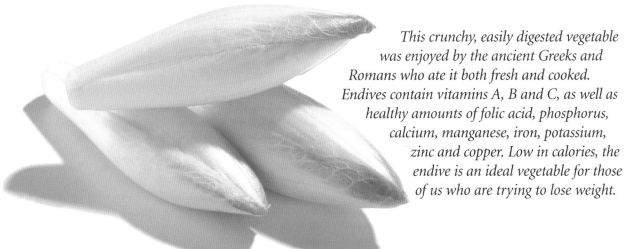

This crunchy, easily digested vegetable was enjoyed by the ancient Greeks and Romans who ate it both fresh and cooked. Endives contain vitamins A, B and C, as well as healthy amounts of folic acid, phosphorus, calcium, manganese, iron, potassium, zinc and copper. Low in calories, the endive is an ideal vegetable for those of us who are trying to lose weight.

Health Benefits

- Aids intestinal function
- Combats gout
- Diuretic
- Stimulates the digestive organs

Put To Good Use

Include endives as a vegetable side dish when eating meat or stews rich in calories; the endive will aid digestion.

Caution

Endives should be eaten young, when still fresh, since they become bitter when exposed to light.

Selecting & Storing

Choose crisp, fresh-looking endives that are free of bruises and blemishes. They should have been stored in the dark, with a lovely white to yellowish color. They will not keep for longer than four days in the vegetable drawer of the refrigerator.

Culinary Use

Raw endive is marvelous in salads, sprinkled with a mustard vinaigrette and garnished with nuts. Steamed, with a pat of butter, cooked endives make a delicate vegetable accompaniment to almost any meal.

Recipe

- Braised Endives (page 180)

Great Combinations

Consider endives with apples, Gruyere cheese and walnuts or hazelnuts. The endives and apples supply fiber, while the cheese and nuts supply calcium. The unsaturated fats of the nuts and the dietary fiber of the fruits and vegetables are particularly good for the cardiovascular system.

Healthful Hints

An endive that is no longer fresh becomes bitter. To get rid of the bitterness, simply use the point of a knife to cut out the cone of the stem which connects to the leaves at the base of the endive.

Good To Know

Endives are a source of important trace elements, notably selenium which protects the cells from aging. Ten percent of our recommended daily amount of selenium can come from a single serving of endive.

Fennel

This green, celery-like vegetable has fine leaves similar to dill with a slight aniseed or licorice flavor. It has medicinal properties of great importance, both to diabetics and to sufferers of rheumatism. Fennel is very rich in vitamins, minerals and iron. It is also rich in beta carotene and folic acid, an important substance for expectant mothers.

Health Benefits

- Appetite stimulant and diuretic
- Combats flatulence
- Heals respiratory inflammation
- Helps prevent anorexia
- Relieves colic and stomach cramps

Home Remedy

Use 1 tsp (5 ml) of fennel seeds, boiled for five minutes then steeped a further 10 minutes, as a tonic to improve digestion.

Caution

Fennel is not recommended for women who are breastfeeding or for children under a year old.

It is not advisable to take fennel on a daily basis for more than two weeks consecutively.

Selecting & Storing

Choose a fennel bulb that is firm without wilted leaves or stalks. It will keep for at least 10 days in a perforated plastic bag in the refrigerator.

Culinary Use

Fennel is as delicious raw as it is cooked; it cooks rather like celery. Use only the bulb, since the stalks are too fibrous. Eaten as is, sliced fennel makes a delicious hors d'oeuvre that tantalizes the appetite and adds a nice crunch to salads. Cooked, the aniseed flavor becomes less pronounced but adds a subtle hint to soups. Cooked fennel is a uniquely flavored vegetable side dish that goes well alongside a variety of meat and fish dishes.

Recipes

- Braised Fennel in Tomato Sauce (page 181)
- Fennel Salad with Orange (page 217)
- Fennel Soup (page 168)

Healthful Hints

Adding chopped fennel stalks to the cooking water for pulses (dried beans or lentils) helps to make them more easily digestible and reduces the chance of flatulence.

Garnish your cheese platter with an arrangement of raw fennel: it will aid in digestion.

Good To Know

In India, roasted fennel seeds are offered after a meal to freshen the breath and help digestion.

F

Fenugreek

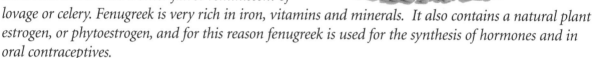

An annual plant that grows to only eight or nine inches (20 cm) in height, fenugreek is one of the oldest known plants cultivated by humans for its use both as a food and as a medicine. It has the aroma of cut hay, while its seeds and leaves have a bitter flavor reminiscent of lovage or celery. Fenugreek is very rich in iron, vitamins and minerals. It also contains a natural plant estrogen, or phytoestrogen, and for this reason fenugreek is used for the synthesis of hormones and in oral contraceptives.

Health Benefits

- Aids in the prevention of hypertension (high blood pressure)
- Combats anemia
- Helps eliminate intestinal worms
- Helps to control glucose levels in diabetics
- Lessens the pain caused by arthrosis (joints) or neuralgia (nerves)
- Lowers blood cholesterol
- Relieves bronchitis, colds and various allergies
- Relieves inflammation

Put To Good Use

A fortifying liquor

Soak 2 oz. (60 g) of fenugreek seeds for 12 hours in ¼ cup (60 ml) of 60 percent proof alcohol. Add 4 cups (1 liter) of white wine and let stand for 10 days. Filter and drink three small glasses per day as a fortifying aperitif.

Caution

Fenugreek seeds have long been used to provoke uterine contractions to help women in childbirth. As a security measure, we do not recommend that pregnant women take any more fenugreek than their usual dietary amount, since this may cause false labor and possibly premature delivery.

Selecting & Storing

As with all spices, fenugreek seeds can be easily stored for several months in a sealed container in a dry, dark place.

Culinary Use

Fenugreek seeds are used in the preparation of stews and curries, and they lend a unique flavor to salads and fish dishes, especially when the seeds have been sprouted.

Recipe

- Indian Split Pea Soup (page 174)

Healthful Hints

The skin on fenugreek seeds is particularly tough: another good reason to soak and germinate the seeds for use as sprouts.

Prepare your own mixtures of spices; this will save you time when you come to cook a meal.

Good To Know

The modern food industry uses fenugreek to create the aroma and taste of maple syrup in a number of food products.

Fig

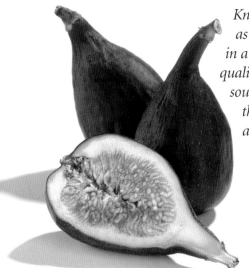

Known for centuries for its therapeutic properties, notably its use as a cancer-fighter, the fig is once again finding a prominent place in a healthy diet thanks to dieticians who recognize its healing qualities. Low in fats and salt, figs are rich in dietary fiber and are a source of calcium, magnesium and potassium. They also contain the rare nutrient vitamin B_6. Fortifying and easily digested, figs are a favorite with athletes.

Health Benefits

- Aids in the prevention of cancer, notably colon cancer
- Combats intestinal irritation
- Lowers blood pressure
- Normalizes cholesterol levels
- Relieves constipation

Home Remedy

Constipation relief

Cut four fresh figs into quarters and cook in a small amount of milk with a handful of raisins. Eat in the morning for breakfast.

Caution

Since figs are rich in sugar, they should be consumed in moderation.

Selecting & Storing

It is often difficult to find good quality fresh figs since they blemish and bruise so easily. However, they can usually be found at specialty grocery stores and at some larger supermarkets. Choose fruit with a pleasing aroma, that are firm and tender at the same time, but do not crush easily. The stem tip should also be firm. Figs keep for only two or three days in the refrigerator. Dried figs can be easily stored for several months in a dry place away from the light.

Culinary Use

Our tendency is to think of figs as a breakfast food (in cereals, porridge, muffins and fruit salads), when in fact they are also truly delectable in spicy meat stews.

Recipes

- Apricot, Fig and Clementine Purée (page 135)
- Bran Fig Muffins (page 141)
- Warm Fig and Apricot Fruit Compote (page 239)

Healthful Hints

Figs tend to be very sticky and somewhat difficult to cut up. To make chopping easier, refrigerate figs for one hour before cutting, or simply run your knife under ice-cold water just before cutting.

Good To Know

Thanks to their very high content of dietary fiber—and in spite of their high sugar content—figs are recommended for overweight people because they stay longer in the stomach, giving a greater sense of fullness, reducing the craving for more food.

F

Fish

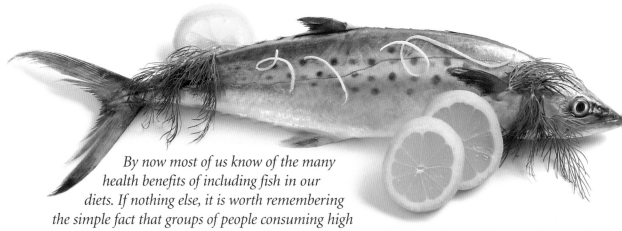

By now most of us know of the many health benefits of including fish in our diets. If nothing else, it is worth remembering the simple fact that groups of people consuming high amounts of fish are rarely affected by heart disease. It is no wonder, then, that health-conscious people include fish as an important element of their everyday diet. Meanwhile, new findings are making an even stronger case for fish: recent studies into the presence of omega-3 fatty acids in fish—notably in so-called "fatty" fish such as herring, mackerel, salmon, tuna and sardines, all of which are high in omega-3 and vitamin B12—are revealing that their oils also help in the relief of stress, anxiety and depression.

Health Benefits

- Aids in regulating heart rhythm
- Helps in the prevention of breast and colon cancer
- Improves humor and combats depression
- Normalizes the functioning of hormones
- Reduces the risk of cardiovascular disease

Put To Good Use

People who consume meat every day of the week would benefit greatly by substituting a few of those meat dishes with fish. To take advantage of the healing properties of omega-3, fatty acids, it is recommended that we eat "fatty" fish at least twice a week.

Caution

Sushi-lovers beware! The consumption of raw fish carries a certain amount of risk, specifically with herring and Atlantic hake that have been known to carry the Anisakis larvae, a common parasite that can cause a severe, chronic reaction.

A recent study on farmed salmon discovered toxic substances proven to be carcinogenic in people who regularly eat farmed fish. The study was considered exaggerated and alarmist by the majority of specialists, who continue to recommend that farmed fish can be safely included in our weekly diets. Farmed salmon now accounts for more than half of the salmon eaten worldwide.

Selecting & Storing

The freshness of fish is the all-important quality that will convince a reluctant fish-eater to give this wonderful, flavorful food another try. Quality fish is generally easy to recognize: the odor should be pleasant and reminiscent of the freshness of the sea, the skin should be rich in color, the flesh should be firm without color near the backbone, and the eyes should be convex with clear brilliant pupils.

Culinary Use

There are dozens of ways to incorporate fish into your diet and, whatever the method, it generally requires very little cooking time. Fish can be grilled, poached, baked, pan-fried or sautéed. Fish makes for an elegant main course or a delicate soup.

Recipes

- Fillet of Raw Salmon with Herb Salt (page 153)
- Pizza with Sockeye Salmon and Fresh Vegetables (page 202)
- Salmon Fillets with Sesame (page 199)
- Salmon Steaks with Green Pepper (page 198)
- Sardine Canapés (page 150)
- Spicy Fish Fillets (page 198)

Healthful Hints

Cooking at high heat can destroy almost half of the precious omega-3 fatty acids in fish. To avoid this, do not hesitate to use the microwave for cooking fish. It will conserve all the nutrients while ensuring the fish is cooked to perfection (see in particular the microwave recipe above for Salmon Steaks with Green Pepper).

Good To Know

Tuna, which we often buy canned, is a less fatty fish, containing only half the omega-3 found in canned Atlantic salmon. Canned sardines and mackerel generally have higher amounts of omega-3 than tuna.

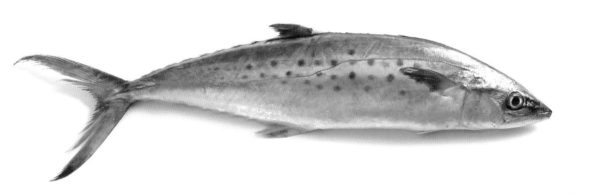

F

Flax

The history of flax (also called linseed) is truly remarkable. For centuries, it was widely used in a variety of products: as a textile fiber to make linen and paper, as a medicine and as an oil for making paint. It was only recently, when the plant was given as a feed to cattle, that the incredible nutritional value of flaxseed for humans was discovered. Flaxseed contains alpha-linolenic acid, a compound that is part of the family of omega-3 fatty acids. In the early 17th century in Quebec one of North America's first farmers, Louis Hebert, brought flax to the New World for the first time. From there, cultivation spread across the continent. Canada is now the world's number one producer of flax.

Health Benefits

- Aids in the prevention of cancer, notably breast, uterine, colon and prostate cancer
- Aids in the prevention of osteoporosis in menopausal women
- Enhances function of the kidneys
- Improves mood
- Increases levels of "good" (HDL) cholesterol
- Lowers levels of "bad" (LDL) cholesterol
- Lowers the risk of cardiovascular disease
- Relieves arthritis

Put To Good Use

Try including two or three tablespoons of ground flaxseed in your daily breakfast cereal, with yogurt or in salads, so as to enjoy all the healing properties of this extraordinary plant.

Caution

As mentioned, to take full advantage of flaxseed, you should first grind the seed since the body's digestive tract is unable to dissolve or break open the seed's hard covering. (Note that boiling or roasting seems to destroy most of the seed's healthy nutrients.)

Flaxseed (linseed) oil is not unanimously praised by nutrition specialists, many of whom argue that the oil contains only a fraction of the seed's lignan, an antioxidant and a plant form of estrogen with healing properties. Since flaxseed oil turns rancid in very little time, it is important to keep it in the refrigerator, and to consume it as soon as possible once the container has been opened.

Flaxseed is not recommended for people suffering from intestinal diverticulitis since the small seeds may get lodged in the membranes and aggravate the condition.

Selecting & Storing

Flaxseed should be bought whole and can be easily stored in a sealed container in the refrigerator.

Culinary Use

Unfortunately, flaxseed added to flour to make cakes, bread or muffins does not actually retain the healthful properties of the flax, since cooking destroys many of the seed's benefits. Nevertheless, it is easy to incorporate flax into your diet by simply adding the ground seeds to breakfast cereals, juices, yogurt or other dairy desserts.

Recipes

- Budwig Cream (page 137)
- Flaxseed Spread (page 154)

Healthful Hints

Soaking flaxseed overnight in a little water will make it easier to digest.

Flaxseed sprouts

You can germinate flaxseed to make sprouts that can be added to salads or used as a garnish for sandwiches. To sprout the seeds, put 2 tbsp (30 ml) of flaxseed into a 1-quart (1-litre) jar. Small seeds like flax should just barely cover the bottom. Cover with non-chlorinated water and leave to soak overnight. The next day, cover the opening of the jar with a piece of cheesecloth or fine plastic mesh, securing it with an elastic band around the mouth of the jar. Pour out the soaking water, rinse well with fresh water and drain. While rinsing one more time before draining, spread out the grains along the inside wall of the jar. Lie the jar on its side on a dark shelf. Rinse two or three times each day.

After two or three days, once the seeds have germinated, place the jar in a sunny place so that the sprouts can develop chlorophyll, an excellent source of vitamin A.

Good To Know

Flaxseed contains 70 percent omega-3 fatty acids—more than avocado and fatty, cold-water wild fish, even though these are rich in alpha-linolenic acid.

In recent years, a number of large egg producers have begun to add flaxseed to the feed given to their laying hens, thereby marketing their eggs as "enriched with omega-3."

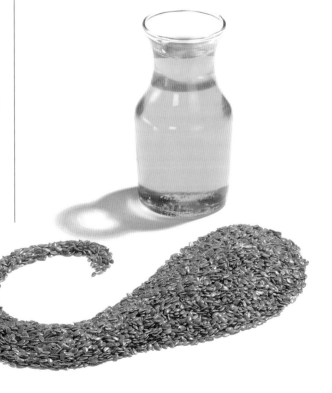

F

Garlic

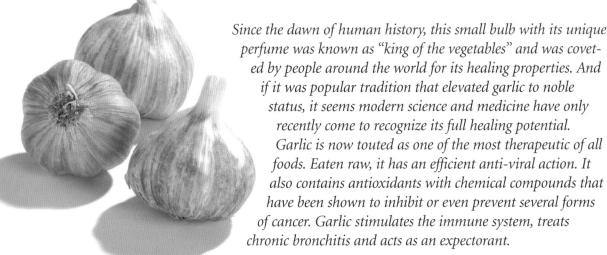

Since the dawn of human history, this small bulb with its unique perfume was known as "king of the vegetables" and was coveted by people around the world for its healing properties. And if it was popular tradition that elevated garlic to noble status, it seems modern science and medicine have only recently come to recognize its full healing potential. Garlic is now touted as one of the most therapeutic of all foods. Eaten raw, it has an efficient anti-viral action. It also contains antioxidants with chemical compounds that have been shown to inhibit or even prevent several forms of cancer. Garlic stimulates the immune system, treats chronic bronchitis and acts as an expectorant.

Health Benefits

- Aids in the prevention of arthritis, relieves arthritic pain
- Aids in the prevention of cancer
- Antiseptic
- Fortifies and invigorates
- Helps eliminate intestinal worms
- Lowers blood pressure
- Stimulates the appetite

Put To Good Use

It is extremely beneficial to eat two large raw cloves of garlic a day. To benefit fully from its antibiotic properties, the peeled clove of garlic should be crushed in a mortar or under a heavy knife, or else minced finely. It can then be added to a salad along with lemon juice instead of vinegar. The simple action of crushing garlic and adding lemon juice liberates ajoene (named after the Spanish word *ajo* for garlic), a compound that is an effective blood thinner.

Caution

Garlic powder possesses very few of the healing properties of fresh garlic and cannot be considered a substitute. Garlic capsules or pills likewise contain very few of the active compounds found in fresh garlic.

Consumed in large amounts, raw garlic can irritate sensitive stomachs and cause heartburn. Garlic is also not recommended for people with dermatosis and herpes-like skin outbreaks or intestinal irritations, and should be eaten in moderation by women who are breastfeeding.

Garlic should not be consumed with sugary foods or milk. It is also not advisable to combine it with hot oil, or deep-fried or starchy foods.

If you want to enjoy the healing benefits of raw garlic, begin slowly, gradually adding more garlic to your diet, and be sure to chew your food well.

Cooked garlic loses it antiviral properties but does retain many of its other benefits. It is therefore highly beneficial to eat some each day, cooked or raw. Garlic is a precious ingredient that heightens the flavors of many dishes.

Indigestion associated with garlic has been linked to the germ inside the clove. It is advisable to remove this greenish sprout inside the garlic clove before consuming.

Selecting & Storing

There are about 300 different varieties of garlic. Regular white garlic is the variety that seems to possess the most properties, both medicinal and culinary. Choose a head of garlic with fleshy cloves that are not sprouting. A head that is dry and falls apart is not fresh. Store garlic in a cool, dark, dry place. In an aerated container, it will keep for several weeks.

Culinary Use

Garlic is a star ingredient in Mediterranean cooking. Gourmets and food enthusiasts from around the world revere garlic for the flavors and aromas it lends to cooked dishes. With the exception of desserts, garlic can be added to almost any dish and it can be cooked in any number of ways.

Recipes

- Aïoli Sauce (page 223)
- Artichokes with Garlic and Lemon (page 149)
- Creamy Garlic and Vegetable Soup (page 166)
- Fresh Tomato Sauce (page 226)
- Harissa Chili Sauce (page 223)
- Pasta Puttanesca (page 202)
- Spinach and Tomato au Gratin (page 152)
- Stuffed Mushrooms (page 152)

Great Combinations

Try combining raw cabbage with fresh garlic to make a potent cocktail of prevention. These foods are both rich in sulfur compounds, known to help in the prevention of many forms of cancer.

Healthful Hints

Controlling garlic breath

As we all know, garlic does not just "perfume" foods; it perfumes whoever eats it! The best way to deal with garlic breath is to chew a few sprigs of parsley or fresh mint leaves after your meal, then rinse your mouth with a mix of water and lemon juice. You can also try chewing on fennel seeds. If the odor persists, take consolation from the fact that your breath is a badge of honor uniting you with other garlic-lovers! And if you've just shared a meal with guests, then you can all regale the virtues of garlic without being offended by each other's breath!

The aroma that won't quit

To get rid of the garlic smell on your fingers, wash fingers in cold water while carefully scraping them with the blade of a stainless steel knife.

Good To Know

The American National Cancer Institute has placed garlic in the number one spot on its list of anti-cancer foods.

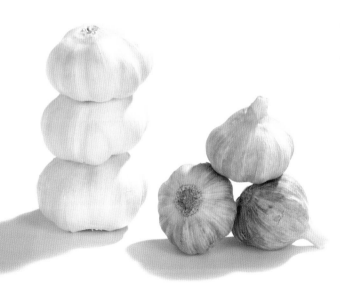

G

Ginger

This root tuber has been used in cooking by Southeast Asians for a few millennia and is reputed to heal a wide variety of infections. In Europe, ginger gained its reputation as a remedy for nausea, specifically in Germany where it was widely used for nausea and motion sickness. It has also proven itself effective in the relief of arthritis, headaches and colds. Our appreciation for this unique seasoning continues to grow as it finds its way into Western cuisine.

Health Benefits

- Aids in the prevention of ulcers
- Anti-coagulant
- Antiseptic
- Calms nausea and helps prevent vomiting
- Combats and relieves arthritic and rheumatic pain
- Combats flatulence
- Fortifies and invigorates
- Relieves headaches and flu and cold symptoms
- Stimulates digestion

Home Remedy

At the first sign of a cold, boil two slices of fresh ginger in a cup (250 ml) of boiling water and steep for 10 minutes. Add a pinch of cinnamon to enhance flavor. This herbal remedy is equally effective for relieving both arthritic pain and stomachache, and in helping digestion.

Caution

Consumed in large amounts, ginger can cause diarrhea. As with all natural food remedies, it is best to practice moderation by introducing a new healing food slowly and progressively into your diet.

Pregnant women can relieve morning sickness by taking ginger. We would recommend, however, that they limit themselves to not more than 1 tsp (5 ml) fresh ginger a day.

Selecting & Storing

Choose ginger roots that are firm and plump with fine, pale silver skin. Rhizomes should be long, the length being a measure of maturity and a sign that they contain more fiber. Ginger can be stored at room temperature and it freezes well, either grated or whole.

Culinary Use

Ginger has a delicate yet spicy flavor that lends itself to a variety of uses: it adds an exotic aroma to soups, the sauces of a main course, vegetable dishes, stews and curries, salad dressings, desserts and hot beverages. It comes in a varitey of forms: fresh, powdered, crystallized, dried, ground and as a syrup or a marmalade. The root's healing properties, however, are most potent when consumed fresh; grating is one of the best ways to release its health-giving compounds.

A Great Combination

The aroma of ginger harmonizes well with coriander, lemon and orange. Add finely cut strips to a vegetable salad. Rich in vitamins, the salad will be low in calories and high in dietary fiber.

Recipes

- Apricot, Fig and Clementine Purée (page 135)
- Beet and Carrot Salad (page 156)
- Cranberry Sauce with Orange and Ginger (page 225)
- Curried Yogurt Dip with Pineapple (page 226)
- Ginger Beer (page 245)
- Green Tea with Ginger and Mint (page 246)
- Indian-Style Braised Cauliflower (page 179)
- Linguine with Almond (page 201)
- Super-Healthy Vinaigrette (page 227)

Healthful Hints

To grate ginger so as to preserve its goodness, peel the root, then crush it with a garlic press.

Ginger can be made into a preserve by maceration (soaking): in a glass canning jar, cover peeled and sliced roots with sherry, vodka or sake.

Beauty Secret

Relax in a soothing bath

Add 2 tbsp (30 ml) of powdered ginger to hot bath water. Do not be alarmed if the skin becomes slightly pink; this will soon disappear.

Gardening Tip

A lovely kitchen plant

Choose a fresh, healthy ginger root and plant in a shallow pot filled with compost and potting soil. Water and place near a sunny window. After about six weeks you should see the first sprouts of a new tropical plant.

Good To Know

Commercially available ginger ale and other drinks contain very little ginger and offer minimal health benefits. You can make your own ginger beer—a stronger-flavored version of ginger ale—by following the recipe on page 245.

When using dried ginger, only one fifth of the measured amount is needed for a recipe calling for fresh ginger. Half an ounce (15 g) of fresh ginger is equivalent to a ¼-inch (7-mm) slice of an average size root.

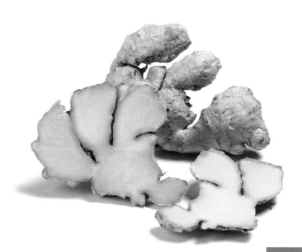

G

Grape

For thousands of years, since prehistoric peoples first began to cultivate the vine of this fruit, the grape has been highly respected for its sweetness as well as its therapeutic benefits. To ancient cultures, the grape often achieved divine status due to the properties of the wine made from it. It is interesting to note that only recently have we discovered the source of the remarkable healing properties of red wine: a powerful antioxidant capable of reducing the risk of cardiovascular disease and cancer. If quercetin (the flavonoid compound of wine) is also found in the grape, it seems that the concentration and fermentation processes of winemaking actually enhance these benefits. In recent decades, research has focused on the healing properties of flavonoids in the grape, particularly resveratrol that is concentrated in the skin of the fruit, and substances called oligomeric proanthocyanidins (OPCs) found in grapeseed.

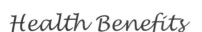

Health Benefits

- Aids in prevention of dental cavities (grape)
- Anti-viral effect
- Combats aging of the skin (grape)
- Fortifies and invigorates
- Laxative
- Lowers blood pressure
- Lowers cholesterol levels (grape, grapeseed, wine)
- Protects against cardiovascular disease (wine)
- Protects against various types of cancer (wine)
- Reduces eye stress associated with bright light
- Relieves hemorrhoids (grape)
- Treats venous insufficiency and varicose veins

Put To Good Use

Red wine should be consumed in moderation so as to benefit from its healing properties; the daily amount should not be more than two glasses.

Caution

Grapes must be carefully washed before eating since their skins may be slightly contaminated with pollutants, pesticide residue or mildew.

The negative health and psychosocial effects of excessive alcohol consumption are well known by most of us. Wine should be consumed in moderation.

Selecting & Storing

Grapes keep well in the refrigerator for about a week, and they can even be frozen for a few weeks.

As for wine, it is well known that fine wines will keep for decades in their unopened bottles, and will improve in flavor over time. Once opened, however, wine deteriorates quickly in contact with air, and a noticeable change in flavor is noticed within a few hours.

Culinary Use

Fresh grapes are one of nature's gifts. They can accompany a platter of raw vegetables or cheeses, or be added to either vegetable or fruit salads. Grapes will amaze you when added to the gravy or sauce of wild game.

Recipes

- Bran Fig Muffins (page 141)
- Brown Rice with Almond and Raisin (page 185)
- Fresh Grape Jam (page 136)
- Homemade Granola (grapeseed oil) (page 139)
- Homemade Muesli (raisins) (page 143)
- Warm Fig and Apricot Fruit Compote (raisins) (page 239)
- Zucchini Chocolate Loaf Cake (grapeseed oil) (page 237)
- Zucchini Buckwheat Loaf Cake (grapeseed oil) (page 238)

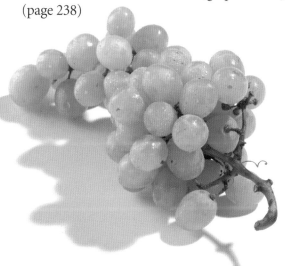

Great Combinations

A salad of couscous or quinoa with parsley (see recipe for Taboulé on page 216), garnished with fresh grapes, is a dish high in micronutrients and low in calories (thanks to the tomato, lemon and fresh mint). It is also full of preventive healing properties since the olive oil supplies the unsaturated fat needed for the protection of the blood vessels.

Healthful Hints

Soak fresh red and green grapes in a little olive oil with a few sprigs of thyme or rosemary and the zest of an orange or lemon. Marinate for one or two hours before piercing and arranging in alternating colors on bamboo skewers. Place on the BBQ or in the oven to grill after you've finished grilling your vegetables, meat or fish.

Grapeseed oil is rich in polyunsaturated fats that will not decompose into toxic compounds when heated to high temperature, making it one of the best oils for cooking.

Beauty Secret

Softens rough skin

Crush a few grapes into liquid honey and apply to the skin. Leave on for 20 minutes, then rinse well and gently pat dry with a towel (without rubbing).

Good To Know

Red wine is far ahead of white wine in terms of healing properties. According to recent studies, red wine contains about twice the number of phenol compounds—and twice the antioxidant properties—as white wine.

It has also been found that one must drink about three times the amount of purple (not clear) grape juice, compared to wine, to have the same health properties—a good number to remember for those who do not drink wine.

G

Grapefruit

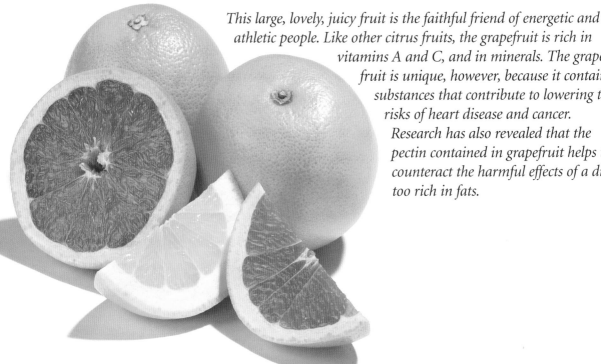

This large, lovely, juicy fruit is the faithful friend of energetic and athletic people. Like other citrus fruits, the grapefruit is rich in vitamins A and C, and in minerals. The grapefruit is unique, however, because it contains substances that contribute to lowering the risks of heart disease and cancer. Research has also revealed that the pectin contained in grapefruit helps to counteract the harmful effects of a diet too rich in fats.

Health Benefits

- Anti-hemorrhagic
- Diuretic and aids digestion
- Nutritious and a good source of energy
- Reduces levels of blood cholesterol
- Reduces the risk of cancer
- Relieves cold symptoms
- Stimulates the appetite

Home Remedies

People who are suffering from—or weakened by—a cold or anemia will derive a number of benefits from drinking a glass of grapefruit juice three times daily before meals.

For people with insomnia, grapefruit juice taken before bed will encourage drowsiness.

Before a large feast or a particularly rich meal, peel and eat a whole pink grapefruit. This will help to avoid the overloading of your arteries.

Caution

A grapefruit and its juice (either fresh or frozen) contain substances that can affect the way the body absorbs and processes some medications. If you are taking medication, avoid consuming grapefruit until you discuss the possible conflicts with your doctor or pharmacist.

A grapefruit that is cut in half so as to scoop out the fruit has fewer healing benefits than a peeled grapefruit eaten in sections. This is because about half of the fruit's pectin is found in the inner peel and membranes.

Selecting & Storing

Choose fruit that are heavy and firm. Keep in mind that pink grapefruit contains more lycopene, an important antioxidant for the human body that neutralizes free radicals. Look for grapefruits with the most pronounced red color inside, such as the Ruby, Ruby Red and Star Ruby varieties.

Culinary Use

Grapefruit complements salads and meats, and, combined with other fruits, can be made into excellent desserts.

Recipe

- Fruit Trio Appetizer (page 137)

Great Combinations

Prepare a delicious appetizer using avocado slices and wedges of grapefruit. The light acidity of the grapefruit is pleasantly contrasted with the rich lipids of the avocado. Season with lime juice and fresh herbs such as basil, coriander and mint.

Healthful Hints

When making homemade grapefruit juice, the acidity of the grapefruit can be neutralized by mixing it with sweeter citrus fruits, like oranges or clementines, or with other fruits.

Blend sections of peeled grapefruit with the juice of two oranges and two clementines. Add about 20 strawberries and blend again.

Beauty Secret

Grapefruit juice from a store generally contains less of the fruit's pulp and pectin, and therefore does not have the same potential for lowering blood cholesterol. To benefit most from this fruit, the whole peeled fruit should be eaten or made into juice, including the membranes that separate its sections.

Pink and red grapefruits do not contain more vitamin C than the white variety, but they do have twice as much beta carotene and lycopene.

Good To Know

The grapefruit diet

In this weight-loss diet, all foods are forbidden except grapefruit. Although it is true that this fruit has very few calories, the idea that the acidity of the grapefruit will simply dissolve body fat is quite incorrect. After a few days on this diet the body becomes accustomed to the lower energy intake so that when a regular diet is resumed, the body very quickly regains all the lost weight.

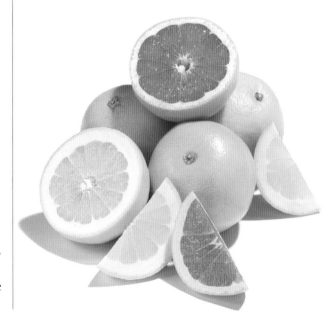

G

Honey

Despite all the therapeutic properties that have been recognized in honey, dating from the most ancient of times, it is today regarded with some reservation by nutritionists. Although honey contains beneficial digestive enzymes and a small number of minerals, its vitamin content is low. The richness of honey is due to the fact that it contains even more sugar than refined white sugar.

Health Benefits

- Aids in the elimination of bacteria
- Combats sore throat
- Relieves cold and flu symptoms
- Relieves constipation
- Relieves the pain of ulcers
- Speeds the healing of wounds

Home Remedy

To relieve a sore throat, mix into a small glass some hot water, the juice of half a lemon and 3 tbsp (45 ml) of honey.

Caution

Never give honey to a young infant since it may contain low levels of the microorganism responsible for botulism.

Also, even though it may contain no artificial flavorings, color or preservatives, honey may include some natural toxins and should be consumed in moderation.

Selecting & Storing

A variety of honeys are available, each with a different color, flavor and aroma depending on the flower from which the bees have made it from. As a rule, the darker the honey, the more flavor it tends to have. It is preferable to eat honey as is, without heating or filtering, to get the most from its therapeutic properties.

Culinary Use

Honey is an excellent replacement for refined white sugar in the preparation of desserts because it is actually lower in calories. Remember to use slightly less honey than sugar since it is sweeter than sugar.

Recipes

- Bananas with Cinnamon and Rum (page 233)
- Ginger Beer (page 245)
- Homemade Granola (page 139)

Beauty Secret

Apply a thin layer of honey to the face before a bath and keep it on throughout. Rinse off with hot water followed by cold water.

Good To Know

Honey is known for its ability to relieve a stomachache. For more acute problems, Manuka honey from New Zealand is shown to be efficient in the treatment of stomach ulcers. After giving 1 tbsp (15 ml) of Manuka honey four times a day to people suffering from ulcers, researchers found that all the patients had relief from their symptoms.

Jerusalem Artichoke

The Jerusalem artichoke, or sunchoke, is a perennial plant with oval tubers that are full of dietary fiber and are one of the best sources of potassium. The lowly appearance of this root crop does it no justice, and so it is rarely seen on our table despite the fact that it originated in North America and was very popular before the advent of the potato.

Fortunately, gourmet chefs are starting to rediscover its delicate artichoke flavor.

Many new mothers will appreciate that Jerusalem artichoke will help them in milk production. Furthermore, people wanting to lose weight will welcome the fact that this tuber contains less starch than the potato, and its slightly sweet flavor will please diabetics, who can eat the Jerusalem artichoke at no risk.

Health Benefits

- Aids in the prevention of high blood pressure
- Excellent energy source
- Promotes milk flow in mothers

Put To Good Use

This root crop is a great substitute for the potato because it contains fewer calories. Adding it to the diet will allow you to benefit from a rich source of potassium.

Caution

This vegetable can cause flatulence in people not used to eating it. The disagreeable effect can be countered by braising the roots instead of boiling them.

Selecting & Storing

Choose Jerusalem artichoke tubers that are firm with unblemished skin.

Culinary Use

Cooked, raw, marinated, baked *au gratin* or whipped, Jerusalem artichoke can be cooked as easily as potato.

Recipes

- Jerusalem Artichoke and Mushrooms (page 183)

Healthful Hints

Plunge peeled and sliced roots into water with some lemon juice to stop them from turning brown.

Good To Know

It is best not to cook Jerusalem artichokes in water since they will lose their nutrients.

As well as for its lower calorie count, people wishing to lose weight should choose this vegetable because it gives a more intense feeling of fullness.

Kiwi

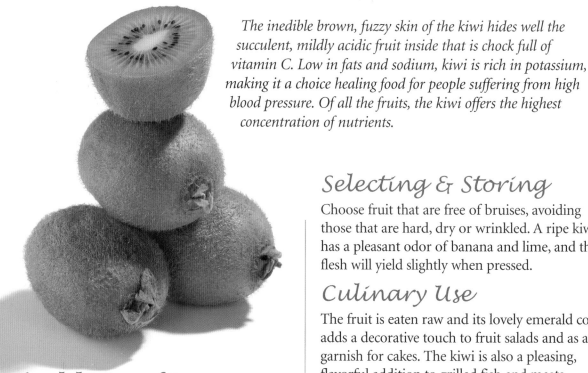

The inedible brown, fuzzy skin of the kiwi hides well the succulent, mildly acidic fruit inside that is chock full of vitamin C. Low in fats and sodium, kiwi is rich in potassium, making it a choice healing food for people suffering from high blood pressure. Of all the fruits, the kiwi offers the highest concentration of nutrients.

Selecting & Storing

Choose fruit that are free of bruises, avoiding those that are hard, dry or wrinkled. A ripe kiwi has a pleasant odor of banana and lime, and the flesh will yield slightly when pressed.

Culinary Use

The fruit is eaten raw and its lovely emerald color adds a decorative touch to fruit salads and as a garnish for cakes. The kiwi is also a pleasing, flavorful addition to grilled fish and meats.

Health Benefits

- Aids in the prevention of cancer
- Combats hypertension (high blood pressure)
- Lowers blood cholesterol
- Relieves cold symptoms

Recipes

- Papaya Shrimp Salad with Kiwi (page 158)
- Summertime Kiwi Smoothie (page 245)

Put To Good Use

Since the kiwi can now be found in supermarkets almost all year round, there is no real reason not to include it in your daily diet. It would be wise to replace that morning glass of orange juice once in a while with a whole kiwi, especially since it contains more vitamin C.

Great Combinations

Create an appetizer with lettuce, diced salmon and slices of kiwi, all sprinkled with a vinaigrette of lemon juice and olive oil. The vitamin C of the kiwi helps the digestion of the iron in the fish.

Healthful Hints

Mix up your flavors by garnishing vegetable or pasta salads with slices of kiwi.

Caution

Kiwis are easily digested by most of us, but people with allergies to papaya and pineapple might also be allergic to kiwi. The reactions may be due to Oral Allergy Syndrome (see entry for Orange on page 86).

Good To Know

When compared weight for weight, the kiwi has more vitamin C than any of the citrus fruits. Just 3 oz. (100 g) of kiwi supplies the recommended daily amount of vitamin C for an adult.

Leek

Along with its cousins garlic and onion, the leek is very rich in minerals and possesses many of the same healing properties. It also contains high levels of folic acid, a form of vitamin B. Low in calories and sodium, it is a must for diabetics and for people on low-sodium diets, as well as for those who want to lose weight.

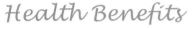

Health Benefits

- Astringent and diuretic
- Helps to destroy bacteria
- Protects against cardiovascular disease

Put To Good Use

Because of its delicate and subtle flavor, the leek pleases the taste buds and offers new healing benefits to those who tend to avoid onions because of their strong flavor.

Caution

Leek can cause flatulence because of its sulfur content. Wash it carefully and thoroughly, removing all of the soil and sand that may have accumulated between its leaves.

Selecting & Storing

Choose a firm vegetable with healthy green leaves. Do not buy leeks that do not have their roots, since these tend to be the ones that get blemished easily. They will keep very well in the refrigerator for at least a week.

Culinary Use

Chopped raw leek lends a delicate flavor to salads. Cooked, it is delicious in soups, baked *au gratin*, in quiches, with rice, or used as a vegetable side dish.

Recipes

- Indian Split Pea Soup (page 174)
- Radish-Leaf Soup (page 172)
- Rice with Leek, Mushroom and Fine Herbs (page 185)
- Sweet Potato and Celeriac Soup (page 171)
- Vegetable Chick-Pea Casserole *au Gratin* (page 196)
- Vegetable, Feta Cheese Quiche with Pecan Crust (page 204)

Healthful Hints

To clean a leek, first be sure to cut off the green part. Then make three or four careful vertical cuts to the stem so as to detach the leaves, before running under cold tap water.

Good To Know

A portion of cooked leek contains almost a third of the daily allowance of folic acid for adults.

L

Lemon

With its invigorating flavor and vibrant yellow color, the lemon owes its health-giving reputation, first and foremost, to its high level of vitamin C. Over the past few centuries, lemons and limes have saved countless sailors from death by scurvy, a terrible disease caused by a vitamin C deficiency that affected many men on long sea voyages. Lemons also contain carotene, minerals and important trace elements. Research has shown that due to its antioxidant properties, the fruit inhibits the growth of cancers and slows the aging process. Its juice and peel are highly valued in the kitchen, and it can also be put to good use elsewhere around the house.

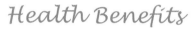

Health Benefits

- Anti-rheumatic, anti-arthritic, treats gout
- Calms and soothes stomach problems
- Helps expel intestinal worms
- Helps prevent colds
- Invigorates and revitalizes
- Restores important minerals to the body
- Treats anemia

Home Remedies

Lemon for colds

At the very first signs of a cold, drink the juice of a freshly squeezed lemon added to hot water. Take several times a day and just before bed.

Two tbsp (30 ml) of freshly squeezed lemon juice in half a glass of water, taken first thing in the morning and just before bed, is an excellent invigorating tonic.

Lemon juice is highly recommended for people with fatigue or those who are recovering from an illness. It is also excellent for children.

Caution

Choose lemons that are ripe. If the peel is to be used (it gives a lovely, fine flavor to salads, salad dressings, meat stews, fish and pasta, as well as to cream sauces and cakes), ensure that the lemon is free of pesticides and preservatives. To maintain its appearance, fruit producers usually coat the fruit in "edible" wax. If you cannot find organically grown lemons, brush the fruits well while washing or leave to soak for a few seconds in boiling water (or several hours in cold water) so as to remove the coating of wax.

As soon as lemon juice comes into contact with the air, the vitamins it contains begin to oxidize and lose their potency. This is also true for the juice of oranges and grapefruits. To obtain the greatest benefit from citrus fruits, try to drink their juice as soon as it is squeezed.

Selecting & Storing

Choose fruit that are firm and ripe with a finely textured peel. As mentioned, choose fruit that have not been treated with chemicals. Store in a cool, dark place.

Culinary Use

Whether cooked or raw, lemon is very useful in the kitchen since the whole fruit is edible. It lends a truly unique flavor to all types of dishes, whether sweet or salty. Each part of the fruit has its own uses. When making salad dressing or vinaigrettes, try replacing vinegar with lemon juice and add in some grated peel. To take best advantage of the fruit's antioxidant properties, add wedges of lemon—including the pith—to fruit or vegetable juices prepared in the blender.

Recipes

- Apricot, Fig and Clementine Purée (page 135)
- Artichokes with Garlic and Lemon (page 149)
- Avocado Dip with Lemon and Anchovy (page 160)
- Fillet of Raw Salmon with Herb Salt (page 153)
- Fresh Beans with Capers and Lemon (page 182)
- Egg-Free Light Mayonnaise (page 224)
- Sparkling Lemonade (page 246)

Great Combinations

Combine olive oil and mustard with lemon (juice and zest) to create a simple, vitamin-rich dressing. For enhanced anti-viral, cold-fighting properties, add minced garlic.

Household Tips

Ink stains on the skin will disappear quickly when rubbed with lemon juice.

To polish copper cookware, rub with slices or wedges of lemon that have been dipped in salt.

Healthful Hints

Before squeezing the juice from a lemon, roll on the counter top applying some pressure with the hand so as to soften the fruit. This will help ensure that the maximum amount of juice gets released when you squeeze it.

If your brown sugar has turned into a solid block from drying out, simply add one or two pieces of lemon peel wrapped loosely in plastic.

Within a day or two the brown sugar will be soft again. Do not allow the peel to come into direct contact with the sugar.

Beauty Secrets

Anti-wrinkle treatment

Apply a mixture of equal parts olive oil and lemon juice to the face and massage gently. The vitamin-rich compounds in the olive oil and lemon have a stimulating effect and will diminish facial wrinkles.

Sparkling smile

A mixture of equal parts (1 tsp / 15 ml) baking soda and lemon juice, used as toothpaste, will brighten the teeth and give a sparkling smile. Rinse the mouth well with water afterwards.

Good To Know

A rounder lemon is generally juicier than an oblong one.

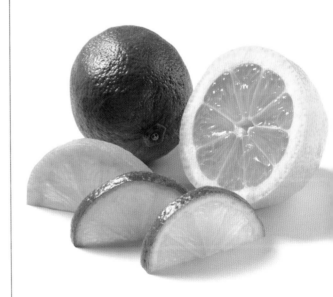

L

Lentils

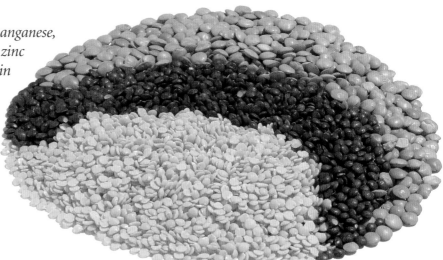

Rich in minerals (calcium, manganese, iron, potassium, phosphorus, zinc and sulfur), lentils also contain vitamin A, some B vitamins (thiamin and riboflavin) and vitamin C. Their high concentration of protein also makes them a 'complete food,' a perfect all-in-one food for manual laborers in particular.

Health Benefits

- Aids in the prevention of cardiovascular disease
- Lowers levels of "bad" (LDL) cholesterol
- Nutritious and aids digestion

Put To Good Use

A serving of lentils is a healthy substitute for a serving of meat since it contains less fat and more fiber. Try to gradually introduce lentils into your diet by substituting ground meat with lentils in spaghetti sauce (see page 208). There is only a slight difference in taste, yet the texture remains rich—and you will feel better for making the change.

Caution

Lentils should be consumed in moderation because of their high concentration of protein and nutrients. This is of particular importance for people with gout.

Selecting & Storing

Brown, green, yellow, orange or red: the choice in lentils is wide. Lentils are easily stored for over six months in a sealed container in a dry, dark place.

Culinary Use

Cooked lentils lend themselves to a variety of uses. They are excellent in salads or soups, or combined with rice or pasta, and they make a healthy side dish alongside a main course with sauce.

Recipes

- Kidney Bean and Lentil Casserole (page 195)
- Lentil Curry with Pistachio (page 193)
- Lentil Soup (page 173)
- Quiche with Millet, Tofu and Lentils (page 203)
- Tagliatelle with Lentil Sauce (page 208)

Healthful Hints

Lentils are the one of the most versatile legumes (pulses). Delicate and pleasing, they cook quickly (in about the same time as rice) and do not require pre-soaking.

Good To Know

The body begins digesting lentils in the mouth. To avoid flatulence, simply chew lentils well.

Lettuce

Among the wide selection of lettuce varieties now available in stores and markets, the most nutritious ones are those with the darkest green leaves. These types contain plenty of carotene and vitamin C, as well as an abundance of minerals and other compounds that combat a variety of diseases. Lettuce contains very little fat, sodium or calories—as long as you limit the amount of salad dressing and seasonings you serve it with. Lettuce is easily digested, contains many vitamins, and possesses benefits that favor sleep for those with insomnia. Endive is recommended for people with jaundice and has fortifying, diuretic, detoxifying and laxative properties. Corn salad (also called mache or lamb's lettuce) is very rich in vitamins, is easy to digest and acts as a gentle laxative. Dandelion greens are an excellent diuretic for people with diabetes, gout or rheumatism.

Health Benefits

- Helps lower arterial pressure
- Helps lower levels of "bad" (LDL) cholesterol
- Helps prevent cardiovascular disease
- Improves blood coagulation
- Lowers the risk of cancer
- Relieves gout and rheumatism

Put To Good Use

To take advantage of the vitamin K in lettuce, a necessary vitamin for the coagulation of the blood, it is recommended that a portion of about 1 cup (250 ml) of lettuce is eaten per day.

Caution

It is best to wash lettuce leaves carefully in several changes of water before eating. However, to take full advantage of their precious healing properties, avoid soaking the leaves.

Despite its popularity, iceberg lettuce contains, unfortunately, very few vitamins and just a lot of water, according to experts.

Selecting & Storing

Choose lettuce with leaves of a rich green color that are crunchy without blemishes. Avoid lettuce with wilted or discolored leaves. Lettuce keeps for about a week in the refrigerator in a perforated

L

plastic bag. Mixed salad greens (mesclun) or spring salad mixtures keep well in sealed containers after being washed, spun and towel dried.

Culinary Use

The possibilities are almost endless for making salads, whether combining different types of lettuce or using one type of lettuce with different kinds of vegetables. Other foods can also be included, such as pasta, legumes (cooked beans, peas or lentils), tofu, nuts and grains, meat, fish, and, of course, fruit. One thing is certain: we must not abuse or over-use prepared salad dressings that are rich in fats. Instead, try to use simple, homemade dressings of yogurt, lemon juice and grapeseed oil, or apple cider vinegar and olive oil. Among the many types of lettuce available, Boston lettuce should be noted for its tender, slightly sweet leaves; Romaine lettuce for its excellent crunch and sweetness; mache (corn salad) and curly endive, both with a light, nutty flavor; curly chicory with its bitter taste; red-leafed radicchio for its crunch and bitterness; escarole with its fleshier, slightly bitter leaves; arugula (rucola or Mediterranean rocket) with its fine spicy flavor; and oakleaf lettuce, mild and tender without bitterness.

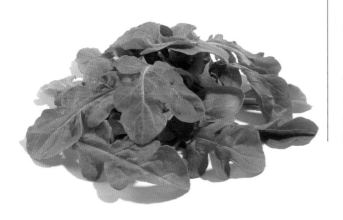

Recipes

- Fennel Salad with Orange (page 217)
- Pear Salad with Pistachio and Chèvre (page 218)
- Salade Niçoise (page 215)
- Strawberry Cantaloupe Avocado Salad (page 157)

Great Combinations

Combine lettuce with calf's liver; the iron of the liver complements the folic acid in the lettuce leaves—two substances that are indispensable for healthy red blood cells.

Healthful Hints

When washing lettuce, add a few drops of white vinegar to the water. This will help to remove any tiny insects that may still be attached.

To preserve the freshness of lettuce over several days, after washing carefully, place in a fairly strong plastic bag with a peeled onion cut in half. Blow up the bag and seal shut.

Keep the wilted leaves of lettuce and add them to soups and soup stocks.

Try to eat some salad every day (the kind that has rich green leaves), especially if it is to replace a meat dish. This is a sure-fire way to achieve radiant health.

Tender young beet and radish leaves can also be combined wonderfully with lettuce.

Good To Know

The rusty-red oxidation that destroys vitamin C can be avoided by tearing lettuce instead of cutting it. Tear it only at the last minute, just before the salad is served.

Mango

With its rich, refreshing flavor, the mango is one of the world's most popular fresh fruits, along with bananas and oranges. There over 500 varieties of this fruit. Rich in beta carotene, vitamins B and C, calcium and potassium, it also has one of the highest concentrations of vitamin A of all fruits.

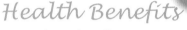

Health Benefits

- Combats skin diseases
- Helps to prevent a variety of cancers
- Lowers the risk of cardiovascular disease
- Slows the aging of cells

Put To Good Use

It is recommended that we eat one or two mangoes each week to keep the body in good health and to preserve the elasticity and softness of the skin.

Caution

Since the skin may cause irritation in the mouth, it is best to peel mangoes before eating: do not use the teeth to separate the flesh from the peel.

Selecting & Storing

A ripe mango has a pleasing odor and dimples when pressed gently with a finger. Avoid fruit that is hard or wrinkled. Do not store in the refrigerator, as mango hates the cold. If it is not yet ripe, leave it to stand at room temperature.

Culinary Use

Mango is at its most flavorful when eaten fresh. Cut into cubes, it complements deliciously a salad of vegetables and fruits, or goes marvelously with shrimp, pork and chicken.

Recipes

- Fruit Cup with Mango Cream (page 234)
- Pineapple Guacamole (page 149)
- Soy Milk with Mango (page 139)

Great Combinations

Drizzle plain yogurt on bite-size pieces of mango. The vitamin-rich mango enhances the yogurt, which is full of calcium and phosphorus. The mango's sweet, mellow flavor requires no added sugar, making it a balanced, light dessert.

Beauty Secret

Crush the flesh of half a mango and apply to the face. Keep this mask on for 30 minutes—while you enjoy eating the other half!

Good To Know

The darker and richer the orange color of the flesh, the higher its vitamin A content.

Millet

Millet is an ancient grain that has been cultivated and consumed by humans for at least 6,000 years and is still the basic foodstuff of many cultures across the world. This cereal has a rich mixture of amino acids and is full of phosphorous, iron, potassium, manganese and niacin. Its high silica content is thought to have a positive effect on blood cholesterol and on the bones.

Health Benefits

- Aids in the prevention of gall stones
- Fortifies and invigorates
- Nutritious energy source
- Regulates the nerves
- Relieves premenstrual discomfort
- Speeds the healing of wounds

Put To Good Use

Women who, for any number of reasons, wish to reduce their consumption of meat would be well advised to add millet to their diet. Thanks to its high concentration of magnesium, millet has a long history of relieving some of the discomfort of the menstrual cycle, and it contains more protein than any other cereal grain.

Caution

Although the risk of allergic reaction is very slight, it has been documented that some people who keep birds in cages have developed serious anaphylactic reactions to eating millet. This grain is the main component of most birdseed, and bird owners have been known to develop a sensitivity to millet dust. This reaction then becomes even stronger by eating millet.

Celiacs (individuals allergic to the gluten of wheat and other grains) are free to eat millet since it is not closely related to wheat, according to the Canadian Celiac Association.

Selecting & Storing

Millet can spoil fairly quickly compared with other grains. It should be stored in a sealed container in a cool, dry place.

Culinary Use

Millet is cooked like rice, at a ratio of 1 cup (250 ml) of millet to 2 ¼ cups (560 ml) of water. It is a better alternative to white rice as a side dish since it contains almost twice as much protein.

Recipes

- Millet Burgers (page 192)
- Millet Casserole (page 182)
- Quiche with Millet, Tofu and Lentils (page 203)

Healthful Hints

When cooking millet, try replacing the cooking water with apple juice. This will give the grain a sweeter, milder and finer flavor.

Good To Know

Ground millet cooks faster than whole millet, but the cooked whole grain contains more health-giving nutrients.

Mushroom

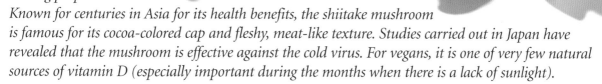

Among the thousands of species of edible mushrooms that have been studied, the shiitake (or Chinese black mushroom) should be noted for its exceptional healing properties.

Known for centuries in Asia for its health benefits, the shiitake mushroom is famous for its cocoa-colored cap and fleshy, meat-like texture. Studies carried out in Japan have revealed that the mushroom is effective against the cold virus. For vegans, it is one of very few natural sources of vitamin D (especially important during the months when there is a lack of sunlight).

Health Benefits

- Aids in slowing tumor growth
- Anti-viral, and combats HIV
- Lowers blood cholesterol
- Stimulates the immune system

Home Remedy

At the first sign of a cold, prepare a soup made from shiitake mushrooms (see page 169). You will enjoy this soup that is also a fortifying cold remedy.

Selecting & Storing

Shiitake mushrooms are sometimes available fresh from Asian food stores or some grocery stores, but it is usually more practical to buy them dried from a health food store.

Culinary Use

Shiitake mushrooms, like most mushrooms, are eaten cooked. They can be bought fresh or dried. To rehydrate dried mushrooms, simply place in a saucepan and cover with water, bring to a boil and simmer for 20 minutes. Before adding to stews or soups, strain, remove stems and chop finely.

Recipes

- Jerusalem Artichoke and Mushrooms (page 183)
- Lentil Curry with Pistachio (page 193)
- Lentil Terrines with Mushroom (page 155)
- Mushroom and Walnut Spread (page 154)
- Mushroom Soup (page 169)
- Spaghetti with Eggplant and Shiitake Mushrooms (page 207)
- Spinach and Mushroom Lasagna (page 200)
- Stuffed Mushrooms (page 152)

Healthful Hints

If you find the flavor of shiitake mushrooms too strong, substitute half the called-for quantity with white or Portobello mushrooms.

Good To Know

Common white (button) mushrooms also contain two vitamins from the B group that are found in few other vegetables: riboflavin (B_2) and niacin (B_3).

Nectarine

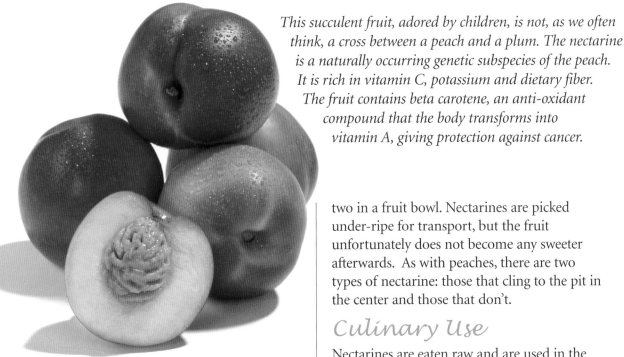

This succulent fruit, adored by children, is not, as we often think, a cross between a peach and a plum. The nectarine is a naturally occurring genetic subspecies of the peach. It is rich in vitamin C, potassium and dietary fiber. The fruit contains beta carotene, an anti-oxidant compound that the body transforms into vitamin A, giving protection against cancer.

Health Benefits

- Helps maintain the immune system
- Helps the body to assimilate iron
- Offers protection against cancer

Put To Good Use

Two ripe nectarines equal more than half the recommended daily amount of vitamin C.

Caution

Some people with hay fever or ragweed allergies may also develop Oral Allergy Syndrome (see entry for Orange on page 86). Stop eating peaches or nectarines if you feel itchiness in the lips and mouth or tightness in the throat.

Selecting & Storing

Choose fruits that are ripe (slightly soft yet still firm) and without blemishes. Store them as you would peaches. Hard fruits will ripen in a day or two in a fruit bowl. Nectarines are picked under-ripe for transport, but the fruit unfortunately does not become any sweeter afterwards. As with peaches, there are two types of nectarine: those that cling to the pit in the center and those that don't.

Culinary Use

Nectarines are eaten raw and are used in the preparation of ice cream, sherbets (sorbets) and pies. They are also a delicious addition to vegetable salads, lending a delicate, rich sweetness.

Recipe

- Yogurt Granola Cup with Nectarine (page 143)

Healthful Hints

Nectarines freeze well. Beforehand, however, be sure to cut them in half, remove the pit and then blanch for two minutes in boiling water with a little lemon juice.

Beauty Secret

Skin cream

As with the flesh of the peach, crushed nectarine applied to the face makes for a rich beauty cream.

Good To Know

Nectarines are richer in vitamin C than their close cousin, the peach.

Nuts

With the exception of peanuts, all of the nuts featured here—Brazil nuts, pecans, almonds, pistachios, hazelnuts and pine nuts— grow on trees. (For walnuts, see page 123.) Almost as rich in protein as meat and fish, nuts can replace animal protein in a number of dishes for a healthy diet. (The amino acids found in nuts, however, are not as well balanced as those in animal protein.) Almonds are rich in vitamin E and fiber; the Brazil nut is rich in saturated fats and selenium, but contains no cholesterol; chestnuts (not shown) have the lowest levels of fats and protein; hazelnuts (also called filberts) are rich in vitamin E and are one of the most digestible nuts; peanuts have the highest protein content; pine nuts, like Brazil nuts, have a high fat content but are very rich in omega-6 fatty acid; and pistachios are very rich in dietary fiber.

Health Benefits

- Aids in the prevention of cardiovascular disease
- Helps the body battle cancer
- Helps the function of the intestines
- Improves health of the bones
- Lowers "bad" (LDL) cholesterol without affecting levels of "good" (HDL) cholesterol

Put To Good Use

A dozen almonds eaten every day as a snack is a good source of magnesium; a mineral that is important for bone formation, the processing of proteins, muscle contraction, the transmission of nerve impulses, the health of the teeth and the health of the immune system. Almonds are also of special interest to menopausal women because they can raise levels of a certain type of estrogen (as well as testosterone) that reduces the amount of bone calcium and magnesium excreted through the urine.

An excellent way to improve your health and enjoy the benefits of nuts is to replace fatty, salty snack foods (like cookies, chips and calorie-rich crackers) with smaller amounts of unsalted nuts.

Caution

High in calories, nuts should be eaten in moderation, preferably to replace fatty foods that have little nutritional value.

Allergens in peanuts and other nuts are the cause of the most common—and most dangerous—of all food allergies. As with other allergies, symptoms of an allergic reaction can begin with itchiness and swelling of the mouth and lips, and a tightening of the breathing passages. This reaction, which in extreme cases is called anaphylactic shock, can cause suffocation and death.

Selecting & Storing

Most nuts are sold in the shell but many can be bought already shelled, roasted, sliced, chopped or ground. Since nuts will go rancid fairly quickly once the shell has been removed, it is best to keep shelled nuts in a sealed container in the refrigerator. Choose nuts that seem heavy for their size, and buy them from stores with a good selection and high turnover of product, to ensure freshness.

Culinary Use

As well as being used for dessert foods like muffins, cookies and cakes, nuts can be used in appetizers, salads, curries and stews, and in side dishes made with rice, couscous and pasta.

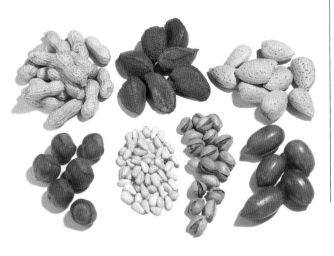

Recipes

- Almond Muffins (page 142)
- Almond (or Walnut) Butter (page 247)
- Brown Rice with Almond and Raisin (page 185)
- Budwig Cream (page 137)
- Cress Salad with Apple, Hazelnut and Chèvre (page 156)
- Lentil Curry with Pistachio (page 193)
- Linguine with Almond (page 201)
- Pear Salad with Pistachio and Chèvre (page 218)
- Quiche with Millet, Tofu and Lentils (page 203)
- Spinach Soup with Pecan (page 170)
- Stuffed Mushrooms (page 152)

Healthful Hints

Make a rich, savory bread coating for fish fillets by blending together pecans and rice or rye crackers, then season with coriander, mint and cumin. Dip fish fillets into beaten egg before covering with the coating. Brown the coated fillets in a pan of oil or clarified butter.

To bring out the full flavor of nuts, they should be roasted. To roast raw shelled nuts, spread them out in a single layer on a cookie sheet and cook for 20 minutes at 350ºF (180ºC). After this time, they should be ready for peeling. The skins of nuts can be removed easily by placing them on a tea towel and gently rubbing until the skins detach.

Good To Know

Nut oils, such as peanut or walnut oil, make for excellent, refined dressings and vinaigrettes.

Oats

A cereal that has enjoyed the biggest boost in popularity in recent years, oats were shown in a study of patients to have reduced their levels of "bad" cholesterol to a spectacular degree. The grain's high concentration of a certain dietary fiber (the gelatin that causes porridge to stick) is believed to be responsible for its health-giving properties. Unlike most other grains that are processed, oat grains are milled without removing the bran and germ, the two parts of the grain where most of the nutrients are found.

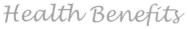
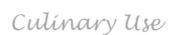

Health Benefits

- Diuretic that reinvigorates
- Excellent source of energy
- Help in the treatment of skin diseases
- Help regulate blood glucose and insulin levels
- Help the body achieve its proper weight
- Lower levels of "bad" (LDL) cholesterol
- Lower the risk of cardiovascular disease
- Promote growth
- Raise levels of "good" (HDL) cholesterol

Put To Good Use

Adding 2.5 oz. (75 g) of oat bran to your diet each day should help lower cholesterol if you have particularly high levels of LDL.

Caution

Oat bran, which contains most of the grain's dietary fiber, is preferable to the whole grain sold as rolled oats.

Selecting & Storing

Oat bran and rolled oats are available in bulk at health food stores and can be stored in a plastic bag on a shelf for several months. In a closed sealed container, oats can be kept for up to a year in the refrigerator.

Culinary Use

Oatmeal porridge cooked in juice or milk makes an excellent breakfast food, while oat bran can be added to soups, meatballs or meatloaf, allowing you to reduce your consumption of meat.

Recipes

- Bran Fig Muffins (page 141)
- Homemade Muesli (page 143)

Beauty Secret

Oat milk for delicate skin

In a small saucepan, bring a glass of water to a boil. Add 1 tbsp (15 ml) of oatmeal and leave to cook for 10 minutes on low heat. Allow to cool, then filter. Add 2 tsp (10 ml) of wheat germ oil and 4 tbsp (60 ml) of cottage cheese. Apply this milk in the morning and evening like a cold cream stored in a dark tinted glass jar, it will keep for about five days.

Good To Know

Finely ground 'instant' rolled oats, though higher in sodium, supply as many vitamins and minerals as coarse-ground oatmeal and oat flakes (which require a longer cooking time).

Olive

The savory fruit of the olive tree is rich in fats and, like the ancient, withered tree itself, seems to be trying to teach us a few secrets about immortality. Olives contain vitamins and minerals in abundance, including calcium and potassium. But it is the oil of the olive that the ancients used and benefited from for many centuries. Recently, various studies conducted in Crete and other regions of the Mediterranean revealed that olive oil can diminish the risks of cardiovascular disease and breast cancer.

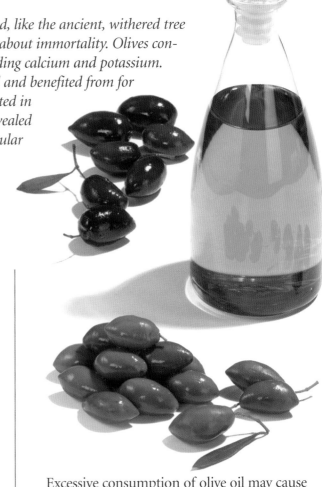

Health Benefits

- Appetite stimulant
- Laxative
- Lowers arterial blood pressure
- Lowers levels of "bad" (LDL) cholesterol
- Protects against cardiovascular disease
- Raises levels of "good" (HDL) cholesterol
- Reduces the risk of breast cancer (olive oil)

Home Remedy

One to 3 tbsp (15 to 45 ml) of extra virgin olive oil (from the first cold pressing), taken on an empty stomach first thing in the morning, helps in the passing of stones, lowers blood pressure and eliminates "bad" (LDL) cholesterol. To slowly ease into this treatment, begin with 1 tbsp (15 ml) of oil per day for several days, before increasing to 2 tbsp, and then finally graduating to 3 tbsp.

Caution

Olives are very rich in salt and should be consumed in moderation, especially by people on a low-sodium diet.

Excessive consumption of olive oil may cause diarrhea. Again, moderation is the best rule to follow.

Individuals who suffer from hemorrhaging should exercise caution in their consumption of olives and olive oil.

Selecting & Storing

Olives are generally sold marinated and can be easily kept in their jars for long periods. Olive oil requires storage away from the light and will keep for only a few weeks. Extra virgin olive oil from cold pressed olives is generally considered to be the highest quality olive oil. The darker the green color, the more pronounced the oil's flavor.

Culinary Use

Black olives found in the market are often green olives that have been harvested before reaching full ripeness. They take on their dark tint during the aging process, after coming into contact with the air or other substances in the marination. Black olives that have been harvested ripe are generally wrinkled.

Whether green or black, olives work beautifully in seasoning and decorating sauces and meat stews, and their rich taste can be recognized in salads and warm or cold hors d'oeuvres. Olive oil—one of the very best cooking oils—is used to prepare delicious salad dressings and vinaigrettes that are highly nutritious for the body.

Recipes

- Braised Fennel in Tomato Sauce (page 181)
- Greek Salad (page 218)
- Pasta Puttanesca (page 202)
- Pizza with Sockeye Salmon and Fresh Vegetables (page 202)
- Salade Niçoise (page 215)
- Vegetable Pasta Salad with Feta (page 217)
- Super-Healthy Vinaigrette (oil) (page 227)

Healthful Hints

Place cubes of chèvre (goat's cheese) in a canning jar, alternating with thyme or other herbs of your choice, and cover with olive oil. Refrigerate for one month before serving as hors d'oeuvres or as an appetizer, or adding to a pasta or green salad.

Beauty Secrets

Did you know that olive oil can slow hair loss? Massage 1 or 2 tbsp (15 to 30 ml) olive oil into the scalp delicately. Cover the hair with a plastic bonnet and a towel for half an hour, then rinse. If you do not like its odor, add a few drops of lavender or jasmine essential oil. Olive oil makes a great makeup remover that also restores moisture to the skin.

Good To Know

A study conducted on 5,000 people in Italy showed that those who regularly consumed olive oil had an average blood pressure rate 3 or 4 points lower than those who consumed less olive oil or consumed butter instead.

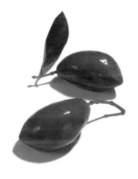

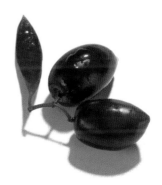

Onion

Since prehistoric times, humanity has marveled and admired the almost infinite healing properties of onions, considered by some as miraculous. This root vegetable remains to this day one of most respected for combating infectious illnesses and for keeping the body in good health. Like its cousin, garlic, the onion is a powerful natural antibiotic. Rich in vitamins and minerals, it also contains a high concentration of sulfur compounds that are known to effectively inhibit the development of cancerous cells.

Health Benefits

- Aids in improving blood flow
- Appetite stimulant
- Decongestant for bronchioles and helps treat respiratory problems
- Helps combat bacterial infections
- Helps inhibit the growth of cancerous cells
- Helps in the prevention of atherosclerosis
- Lowers and stabilizes the level of blood sugars
- Lowers levels of "bad" (LDL) cholesterol
- Promotes hair growth
- Reduces inflammation
- Slows coagulation (blood clotting)
- Stimulates and raises levels of "good" (HDL) cholesterol

Put To Good Use

Onion should be eaten every day. At the top of its list of benefits, just half a raw onion will successfully raise the level of "good" (HDL) cholesterol in the blood by 30 percent. A tablespoon of cooked onion taken at the end of a meal rich in fats will help stop the blood from thickening. Note that the therapeutic properties of the onion are at their best when the vegetable is eaten raw.

Home Remedies

Liquid cold remedy

Boil three onions that have been sliced but not peeled in 1 quart (1 litre) of water for 15 minutes. Filter, cool and store in the refrigerator. Drink one glass upon waking in the morning and one before bed at night.

Syrup for a sore throat

Boil 3 oz (100 g) chopped onion in 1 cup (250 ml) of water for five to 10 minutes. Filter, then add 1 tbsp (15 ml) of honey and stir until the mixture has the consistency of a thick syrup. Take 4 to 6 tsp (20 to 30 ml) each day.

Poultice to relieve minor burns

Mix vegetable oil with cooked onion and apply to a burn.

Caution

Onions are a food with very few negative effects, though they have been known to cause migraine headaches among certain sensitive people.

Selecting & Storing

A number of onion varieties are available: sweet onion, Spanish onion, red onion and white onion. Choose onions that are not sprouting. Most onions will keep for several weeks in a cool, dry place away from the light. They do not require refrigeration.

Culinary Use

The onion, like the other members of its family (green onion, shallot, spring onion and garlic), is a food that lends all of its flavors and nutrients to a multitude of dishes. The green onion is the bulb of a yellow onion harvested well before it has matured, while the shallot is distinguished by its finer taste. Try to imagine the taste of broths and soups without the flavorful onion; likewise salads and salad dressings, marinades, pasta sauces, meat loaf, meat dishes in sauces, casseroles, and stews.

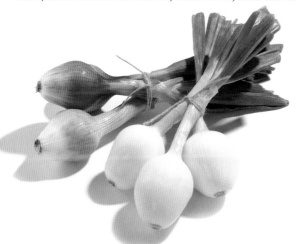

Recipes

- Broccoli Soup (page 167)
- Eggplant Chili (page 197)
- Lentil Soup (page 173)
- Millet Casserole (page 182)
- Onion Soup with Dulse (page 172)
- Parsnip and Zucchini Soup (page 169)
- Ratatouille Niçoise (page 155)
- Tagliatelle with Lentil Sauce (page 208)

Great Combinations

Classic French onion soup is covered with cheese and croutons and is heated in the broiler until the cheese just begins to bubble. This delicious combination provides calcium (from the cheese), complex carbohydrates (the bread), and fructosan from the onion, which gives the soup a diuretic property.

Household Tip

To clean kitchen knives and remove rust, simply rub carefully with a piece of onion.

Good To Know

Some 44 million tons of onions are produced annually in the world, placing it in second place in the rank of cultivated vegetables, just behind the tomato.

Research scientists in Greece have recently found that the onion loses many of its antioxidant properties through cooking.

The shallot contains some unique medicinal properties. A single tablespoon (15 ml) of minced shallot contains a strong dose of vitamin A that fortifies the immune system while at the same time protects the body against eyesight trouble associated with aging, such as cataracts and nyctalopia (poor night vision).

Orange

Is it because the orange is round and has the color of the sun that this juicy, delicious fruit contains so many life-giving properties? As we all know, the orange is a wonderful source of vitamin C, an acid with so many medicinal and health-giving properties, including the ability to fight bacterial and viral infections. Furthermore, in addition to fighting colds and the flu, the orange contains other complex compounds that are effective in helping to prevent cardiovascular disease and inhibiting certain types of cancer.

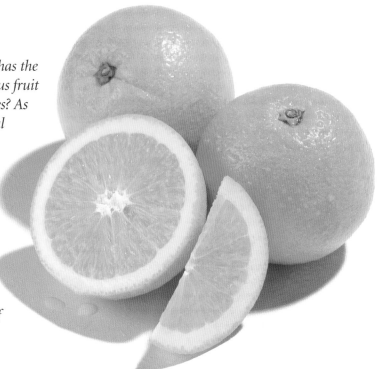

Health Benefits

- Antibiotic and anti-viral
- Anti-hemorrhagic
- Appetite stimulant and fortifier
- Combats different types of cancer
- Lowers the risk of stroke
- Protects vascular tissues
- Purifies the blood
- Reinforces the body's natural defenses
- Rejuvenates cells, especially of the skin
- Relieves asthma
- Relieves rheumatic diseases

Put To Good Use

Drinking a glass of freshly squeezed orange juice each day makes for a potent protection against a number of infections. The juice contains as much vitamin C as the fruit itself, as long as it is taken immediately after squeezing. Contact with air causes the vitamin C content to be lost over time.

The daily consumption of oranges fortifies the whole body, purifies the blood and acts like an internal antiseptic.

To benefit from the cardiovascular protection qualities of an orange, eat the whole peeled fruit, including its pulp and membranes, since these contain the fruit's pectin, the source of many protective compounds.

Caution

Oranges can provoke an allergic reaction known as Oral Allergy Syndrome. It begins with a burning or itching sensation on the lips and mouth, and tightness in the throat. Hay fever and other pollen allergies trigger this increasingly common syndrome, and one can develop allergies to a number of different fruits, vegetables and some nuts as a result. The symptoms disappear quickly after a person stops eating the orange (or other offending food).

Selecting & Storing

The oranges most commonly found in North America come from Florida and California. They will keep for over a week at room temperature—even longer if stored in a perforated plastic bag in the refrigerator.

Culinary Use

The orange is a fruit that serves just as well in a main course as for dessert. Oranges can be cut into thin slices or segmented by hand for green salads, added to pies, creams, sherbet (sorbet) and cakes. Orange juice is also used to add delicious aromas to stir-fried, simmered or sautéed dishes composed of meat or fish, grilled foods, rice and couscous, marinades and salad dressings. The shredded peel and zest also lend themselves to this wide assortment of dishes.

Recipes

- Apricot, Fig and Clementine Purée (page 135)
- Asparagus in Curry Sauce à l'Orange (page 150)
- Cabbage Salad with Spinach, Clementine and Sesame (page 215)
- Cranberry Sauce with Orange and Ginger (page 225)
- Fennel Salad with Orange (page 217)
- Fresh Orange Icing (page 238)
- Fruit Trio Appetizer (page 137)
- Linguine with Almond (page 201)
- Orange and Cherry Soy Smoothie (page 135)

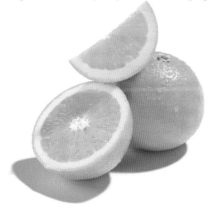

Great Combinations

Prepare a simple, health-giving fruit salad of oranges, bananas and dates. The orange provides vitamin C, while the dates and bananas supply a complement of carbohydrates, fiber and magnesium.

Healthful Hints

To make the peeling of an orange easier, soak for a few minutes in boiling water (off the heat).

Beauty Secret

As with the strawberry, peach, cantaloupe and mango, the orange contains substances that help diminish lines and inhibit wrinkles. Apply a few slices of orange to the face for 15 to 20 minutes before bed each night to help restore the skin's health and add radiance.

Household Tips

To restore the shine to leather handbags or shoes, rub with the peel of an orange, then rub clean with a soft cloth.

Place an orange studded with cloves in a clothes chest or wardrobe to protect garments and woolens from moths.

A few orange peels put into a hot oven after baking (with the oven turned off) will add a lovely scent to the room.

Good To Know

Commercially processed orange juice does not supply the same number of healing properties as freshly squeezed juice. Recent studies have shown that orange juice from the supermarket is almost devoid of its anti-viral compounds.

Papaya

The juicy, sweet flesh of the papaya fruit, which looks like a cross between a cantaloupe and a watermelon, is particularly rich in vitamins A, B and C, in minerals, and in beta carotene. The fruit is also well known as an aid for digestion due to a unique substance it contains: papain. This compound from the papaya has been used for centuries as a natural meat tenderizer, and more recently for digestive medications and ointments.

Health Benefits

- Aids in digestion
- Helps tone the skin
- Lowers the risk of cardiovascular disease

Put To Good Use

For the elderly, or for individuals weakened by illness, the nutritious and health-giving properties of the papaya are particularly appreciated because its soft, tender flesh is so easy to swallow.

Cooked or raw, mixed with other refreshing fruits, it makes for an excellent appetizer.

Caution

The ripe fruit of the papaya has a tender flesh that almost melts in the mouth, with no negative effects in most people. However, people with Oral Allergy Syndrome (see entry for Orange on page 86), should try it in small quantities at first and check for an allergic reaction.

People with a sensitive digestive tract often prefer eating papaya as a fruit sauce, after first puréeing it a blender.

Selecting & Storing

Papaya is ripe when it is slightly soft to the touch. If it needs to ripen further, keep it in a fruit bowl at room temperature for a day or two. To speed up ripening, simply wrap in a brown paper bag, as for an avocado.

Culinary Use

Papaya is usually eaten raw like melon. However, when it is still green, it can be boiled or cooked in fruit juice and served as a fruit sauce.

Recipes

- Papaya Shrimp Salad with Kiwi (page 158)

Healthful Hints

The black seeds at the center of the papaya have a pleasant peppery flavor and can be used as a substitute for capers. To preserve papaya seeds, simply place in a jar and cover with apple cider vinegar, seal the jar and refrigerate. The seeds can also be dried, crushed and ground, later to be used as a seasoning like black pepper.

Good To Know

Papain, the milky substance found in the papaya fruit, has long been used by South Americans to tenderize meat before cooking.

Parsley

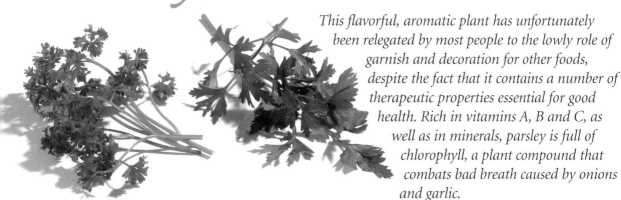

This flavorful, aromatic plant has unfortunately been relegated by most people to the lowly role of garnish and decoration for other foods, despite the fact that it contains a number of therapeutic properties essential for good health. Rich in vitamins A, B and C, as well as in minerals, parsley is full of chlorophyll, a plant compound that combats bad breath caused by onions and garlic.

Health Benefits

- Aids in the prevention of cancer
- Antiseptic
- Combats anemia
- Freshens the breath
- Helps eliminate intestinal worms
- Helps prevent flatulence
- Relieves menstrual discomforts

Put To Good Use

Since it contains antiseptic properties as well as dietary nutrients, raw parsley should be eaten every day, whether in salads or appetizers. This herb provides protection against infections and different forms of cancer.

Caution

Pregnant women should be very careful not to over-consume parsley since it contains substances that stimulate uterine contractions.

Selecting & Storing

Choose curly or flat-leaf Italian parsley, both of which are commonly sold in most grocery stores. Italian parsley is more flavorful in cooking while curly parsley is more attractive for decoration. Both keep well in the refrigerator as long as bunches are kept fresh and dry. As soon as leaves begin to get damp or turn yellow, they should be removed from the bunch and discarded.

Culinary Use

Raw, the leaves and stems chopped fine add flavor and aroma to dressings and give a crunch to salads and cold appetizers. The minced herb can also be used to enhance stews, gravies for a main course and pasta or rice dishes.

Recipes

- Couscous and Parsley Salad (Taboulé) (page 216)
- Super-Healthy Vinaigrette (page 227)

Healthful Hints

Try preparing a salad of green lentils and sprinkle with a dressing seasoned with chopped parsley. The vitamin C in the parsley helps the body to assimilate the iron in the lentils.

Beauty Secret

Skin lotion and hair rinse

Boil a handful of chopped parsley in 1 cup (250 ml) of water until the liquid turns green. Leave to cool, then filter. Use on the skin or as a hair rinse.

Good To Know

One ounce (30 g) of fresh parsley contains 50 mg of vitamin C, or about 80 percent of the daily recommended amount.

P

Parsnip

This root crop is the cousin of both parsley and the carrot, and has a mildly sweet flavor. Its lowly appearance hides a treasure trove of nutrients. Low in calories, the parsnip is rich in minerals and insoluble fiber, making it a perfect vegetable for people who are struggling to control their weight.

Health Benefits

- Aids digestion
- Lowers the risk of colon cancer
- Offers protection against congenital (fetal) malformations
- Relieves bouts of rheumatism

Put To Good Use

A soup of parsnip, leek and onion is a great way to benefit from the healing properties of these three vegetables, all of which are excellent for fortifying the body and offering protection against cancer.

Caution

The over-consumption of parsnip—a very rare situation due the vegetable's unpopularity!—can cause a build-up of coumarin in the body, a compound formerly used as a flavoring that is now banned. In high enough doses, it makes the skin extremely sensitive to sunlight and is toxic to the liver and kidneys.

Selecting & Storing

Choose roots that are firm but not too large, smooth and free of blemishes. With the leaves and stems removed, parsnips will keep for about two weeks in the refrigerator in a perforated plastic bag.

Culinary Use

Raw or cooked, parsnip is used like carrot to make crunchy crudités appetizers, and it adds aroma to soups, mashed potatoes and stews. To benefit most from the root's healing properties, avoid peeling it until it has cooked thoroughly.

Recipes

- Carrots and Parsnips with Dulse (page 151)
- Parsnip and Zucchini Soup (page 169)
- Plantains with Parsnip and Coriander (page 183)

Healthful Hints

Parsnips are better tasting if picked after the first frost since the cold converts some of its starches to sugar. Also, the longer parsnips are stored, the milder their flavor becomes.

Good To Know

A portion of 5 oz. (150 g) of parsnip contains 400 mg of potassium, or 16 percent of the recommended daily amount.

Pea

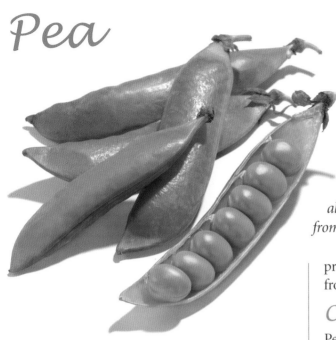

The pea plant belongs to the legume family, the group that includes beans, soybeans, lentils and alfalfa. Fresh peas are rich in vitamins and minerals, and they contain a powerful substance called lutein that gives the vegetable its rich green color. Lutein is highly beneficial for the eyesight and is also an antioxidant that helps stop healthy cells from becoming cancerous.

Health Benefits

- Good source of energy
- Helps intestinal function
- Helps lower levels of "bad" (LDL) cholesterol
- Helps prevent eye cataracts
- Lowers the risk of cancer
- Relieves cold symptoms

Put To Good Use

Even though research has not yet determined the exact quantity of green peas that we should eat to take advantage of the lutein and chlorophyllin they contain—both being known cancer-fighting compounds—it is recommended that we include them as often as possible in our meals, along with other vegetables of the same color.

Caution

Since peas are considered the 'street sweepers' of the intestines, they are not recommended for people with enteritis or intestinal inflammation.

Selecting & Storing

Although fresh peas are generally available only for a few months each year, all of the health-giving properties can be enjoyed year round thanks to the frozen variety.

Culinary Use

Peas are used in soups, stews, and as a common side dish for meat and fish.

Recipe

- Fresh Green Pea Soup (page 173)

Great Combinations

A mixture of green peas and carrots is a traditional favorite and, from a dietary point of view, the fiber in the peas is tempered by the presence of the carrots, making the dish gentler and more digestible. The peas offer a healthy amount of vitamin E while the carrots contribute carotene: two potent antioxidants that work well together.

Healthful Hints

When fresh peas are puréed, they lose a large amount of their dietary fiber component, though this improves digestibility.

Good To Know

Canned green peas lose considerable nutritional and therapeutic value during processing, but they do retain lutein, a substance which helps to prevent cataracts. Frozen peas retain virtually all the health-giving properties of fresh peas, including the vitamin C content.

P

Peach

With its juicy, sweet flesh and lovely aroma, the peach is rich in vitamin A, minerals and beta carotene. Tender and low in calories, the fruit contains a healthy amount of dietary fiber and is easy to digest.

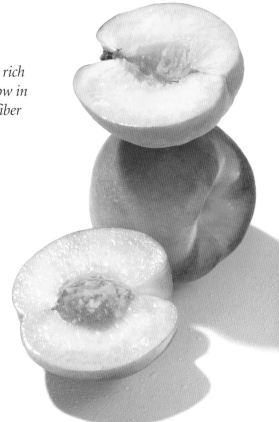

Health Benefits

- Aids intestinal function
- Easily digested
- Fortifying and invigorating
- Offers protection against cardiovascular disease

Put To Good Use

Replace a packaged, high-calorie granola bar with a ripe peach for a snack that is sweet and satisfying—as well as healthier and lower in calories!

Caution

Peaches are often sprayed with a fine coating of edible wax to preserve their freshness. If you are eating the fruit with the peel, wash it carefully just before eating. Consider buying organically grown peaches.

If you experience itching in the mouth or a tightening in the throat from eating peaches, you may have Oral Allergy Syndrome (see entry for Orange on page 86).

Selecting & Storing

Choose peaches that smell good, are not too hard and are free of bruises and blemishes. After picking, peaches continue to ripen and develop their aroma. To speed up the ripening, put peaches in a paper bag that already contains one ripe fruit.

Culinary Use

Peaches are most delicious raw but they can also be cooked. To peel easily, blanch for 30 seconds in boiling water, then place in cold water.

To make a healthy peach milkshake, mix 1 cup (250 ml) soy milk with two chopped peaches in a blender. Add 1 tbsp (15 ml) of honey and a pinch of nutmeg. To thicken further, add 2 or 3 tbsp (30 to 45 ml) of plain yogurt.

Recipe

- Curried Fruits (page 236)

Great Combinations

Add bite-size pieces of fresh peach to spinach, sprinkle with a little coriander and serve with a yogurt dressing. Low in calories, this appetizer is a great source of vitamins and calcium.

Beauty Secret

The crushed flesh of a peach has long been used to preserve healthy skin, keeping it free of wrinkles. Keep the mask on the face for about 20 minutes before rinsing off with warm water.

Good To Know

Canned peaches lose about 80 percent of their original vitamin C content. Bathed in sweet syrup, they also become much higher in calories.

Pear

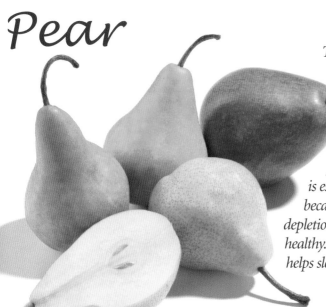

This delectable fruit has a weatlh of nutrients, minerals and B vitamins. The pear also contains lignin, an insoluble dietary fiber that helps lower "bad" (LDL) cholesterol level. Pear can be included in the diet of diabetics—as can most other tree fruits—because it contains fructose, a form of sugar that is not dangerous. Pear is especially recommended for menopausal women because it contains the trace element boron that slows the depletion of calcium from bones, keeping a woman's bones healthy. Boron also stimulates the intellectual faculties and helps slow memory loss associated with aging.

Health Benefits

- Lowers levels of "bad" (LDL) cholesterol
- Lowers the risk of colon cancer
- Stimulates the brain

Put To Good Use

Since pears are now available most months of the year, we would be unwise to stay away from this delicious fruit that contains so many health-giving properties. You only need to eat two pears to obtain 32 percent of the daily recommended amount of dietary fiber. As an added bonus, pears have a reputation for clearing up the complexion and giving soft, glowing skin to those who eat the fruit on a regular basis.

Caution

Since most of the dietary fiber of pears is found in the skin, it is strongly advisable to eat pear with the peel left on (after washing it well).

If you experience itching in the mouth or a tightening in the throat from eating pears, you may have Oral Allergy Syndrome (see entry for Orange on page 86).

Selecting & Storing

Several hundred varieties of pear exist in the world. Those most common in our markets are the Anjou, Bartlett, Bosc and Comice varieties. Rather like the avocado, the pear does not ripen well on the tree but rather develops its fine flavors only after being picked. It then ripens in one or two days before becoming starchy and spoiling quickly.

Culinary Use

Raw or cooked, pears are included in salads, hors-d'oeuvres, and, of course, desserts.

Recettes

- Apple, Pear and Prune Purée (page 136)
- Pear Salad with Pistachio and Chèvre (page 218)

Healthful Hints

To know whether or not a pear is ripe, simply feel where the stem meets the fruit. This spot should be very slightly soft to the touch.

Good To Know

Canned pears retain very few of the nutrients of the fresh fruit. Bathed in sweet syrup, they also become much higher in calories.

P

Pepper, Chili

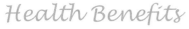

With so many varieties and colors of sweet peppers and spicy chili peppers available, it is no wonder that some people are confused as to which is which…until, of course, they taste them: hot chili peppers then make their presence known! The powerful spiciness of the chili pepper comes from the compound capsaicin that generates a burning sensation on the mucus membranes of the mouth and acts like a decongestant. A chili pepper contains more vitamin C than an orange, but since we eat so little, we do not obtain from it much of our daily requirement.

Health Benefits

- Decongestant for lungs and sinuses
- Helps to prevent bronchitis
- Helps to prevent some types of cancer
- Lessens the intensity of pain
- Lowers blood cholesterol levels
- Lowers blood pressure
- Lowers the risk of cardiovascular disease
- Stimulates the secretion of endorphins

Put To Good Use

To help in preventing chronic bronchitis and colds, drink a glass of water into which 10 to 20 drops of hot chili sauce have been diluted.

Caution

Spicy peppers may increase the acidity of the stomach and irritate the digestive tract, especially in the anus. Experts still do not agree on the effect of chili spice on stomach ulcers: some claim it aggravates and intensifies the pain, while others insist it does the opposite. It is best to exercise caution and eat only a tiny amount, checking carefully for any reaction.

Selecting & Storing

Fresh chili peppers keep well in the refrigerator, but dried and crushed peppers contain all of the same therapeutic properties. Since dried chilis go stale easily, keep them in the refrigerator also.

Culinary Use

The jalapeno, a green chili pepper about the size of a finger, has a flavor that can vary from one fruit to the next. It is used along with its spicy red cousins in broths and soups, in dressings and marinades, in sauces and stews.

Recipes

- Eggplant Chili (page 197)
- Harissa Chili Sauce (page 223)
- Tofu Chili (page 197)

Healthful Hints

Because hot peppers will irritate the skin and eyes, it is best to wear gloves when handling them, or else to wash the hands well with soap several times after handling.

Good To Know

Dried peppers are generally hotter than fresh peppers. Smaller peppers contain more seeds and membranes (where the hot spice is found) than larger peppers, so they tend to be hotter.

Pepper, Sweet

Along with the eggplant and tomato—also in the nightshade family—the sweet pepper is considered, botanically, to be a fruit. Green peppers (not shown) are in fact sweet red peppers that are not fully ripe. Very rich in vitamin C and beta carotene, sweet red peppers contain only small amounts of minerals and B vitamins. Keeping in mind that vitamin C and beta carotene help prevent cataracts, elderly people should ensure that sweet peppers are a regular part of their diet.

Health Benefits

- Fortifies the immune system
- Helps prevent cataracts
- Reduces the risk of cardiovascular disease

Put To Good Use

Added raw to salads twice a week, sweet red pepper boosts the immune system and protects the body against infections.

Caution

Since green bell peppers are actually red peppers that have reached full size but are not fully ripe, they are difficult for some people to digest.

Also, vitamin C, a powerful antioxidant, does not tolerate cooking. To benefit from the vitamin C in sweet peppers, it is best to eat them raw.

Selecting & Storing

Choose red, yellow, green or even purple peppers, all of which keep well in the refrigerator.

Culinary Use

Raw peppers give a pleasing crunch to salads, while cooked peppers add color, aroma and richness to soups, rice dishes, chili sauces and stews. While fried peppers are tasty, grilled or barbecued peppers are more nutritious.

Recipes

- Corn and Quinoa Soup (page 174)
- Ratatouille Niçoise (page 155)
- Sautéed Brussels Sprouts (page 180)
- Spaghetti with Eggplant and Shiitake Mushrooms (page 207)

Healthful Hints

A good way to take advantage of all the healing properties of the sweet pepper is to consume its juice, mixing it with the juice of other vegetables such as carrot, celery and parsnip.

Grilled sweet peppers are another delicious, healthy option. Simply cut peppers in half, place on a cooking sheet with the rounded side upwards and broil until the skin just begins to blacken. Allow to cool, remove blackened parts, inner core and seeds, and add to other cooked dishes.

Good To Know

A sweet red pepper contains three times the amount of vitamin C found in an orange of equal weight.

P

Pineapple

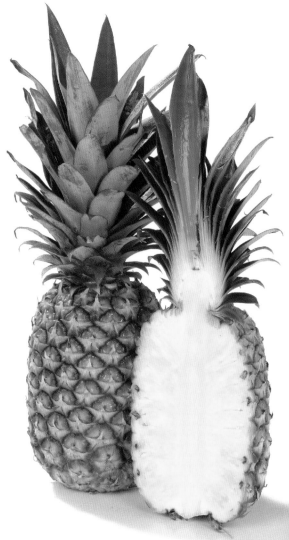

We should not let the thick, rough peel of the pineapple discourage us from eating this sweet, juicy fruit, though King Louis XIV of France is said to have broken his teeth on one! The pineapple is rich in vitamin C, beta carotene, potassium, manganese (an important trace mineral we still do not full understand) and brome-lain, an enzyme complex that can decompose proteins, aid in digestion and relieve arthritic pain. On top of all this, pineapple helps relieve indigestion caused by poor eating habits, such as eating too quickly or not chewing sufficiently.

Health Benefits

- Aids digestion and cleans digestive tract
- Antioxidants that protect against cancer and hardening of the arteries
- Antiseptic and anti-inflammatory
- Combats cellulite
- Diuretic
- Relieves sore throat and cold symptoms
- Soothes some types of heart burn and indigestion

Home Remedy

People with delicate stomachs are advised to eat two slices of pineapple daily, at breakfast or before meals. The same treatment is recommended for people suffering from rheumatic pain. Bottled pineapple juice, due to its high vitamin C content, is highly recommended for people prone to colds.

For quick relief from the pain of a sore throat, gargle with cold pineapple juice.

Caution

The bromelain compound in pineapple that helps prevent indigestion is lost in canning and juice production. To benefit from this healing property, always eat fresh pineapple.

Selecting & Storing

The pineapple is one of a few fruits that stop ripening when harvested; therefore aim to select a ripe, heavy fruit with a pleasing aroma at the base, with leaves that are a healthy green color. Avoid buying discolored fruit or those with a soft peel. The leaves of a ripe fruit will detach with little effort, while the leaves of an under-ripe fruit will be more difficult to remove. Once peeled and chopped, pineapple will keep for a few days in the refrigerator. In some supermarkets, it is sold freshly peeled.

Culinary Use

Served in slices or chunks, eaten as is or mixed with yogurt, pineapple makes a simple, refreshing dessert. The fruit makes a salad succulent, especially when combined with vegetables like spinach and avocado.

Recipes

- Curried Yogurt Dip with Pineapple (page 226)
- Pineapple Guacamole (page 149)

Great Combinations

Use broccoli, sweet peppers and pineapple in an Asian-style stir-fry. All three supply vitamin C and beta carotene, while the pineapple adds balanced carbohydrates and fruit sugars.

Healthful Hints

To make a pineapple sweeten to its best, stand it upside-down for at least twelve hours before peeling.

Beauty Secrets

Clearer skin

Applied externally, pineapple juice is an excellent tonic for healthy skin.

Wart remedy

Rub the wart with a piece of fresh pineapple for a minute or so. Repeat twice daily (morning and evening) until the wart disappears.

Good To Know

By virtue of the bromelain it contains (an enzyme complex that breaks down protein), pineapple is excellent in marinades to tenderize meats and poultry before grilling. Note that just 4 oz. (120 g) of pineapple contains 100 mg of bromelain.

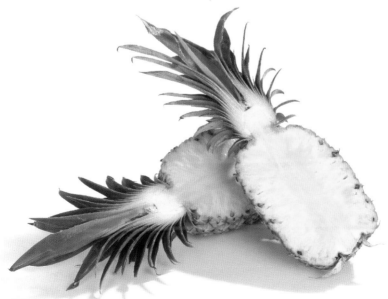

P

Plantain

Resembling its sweeter cousin the banana in shape, the plantain is larger with a green color that tends to be blackish. Treated as a vegetable, it differs from the banana by its coarser flesh and its nutritional content: it is high in vitamin A, does not contain sugar and has more potassium, magnesium and soluble fiber. Because it is rich in starch, it has to be eaten cooked. This starch is transformed into sugars according to the ripeness of the plantain: a yellow fruit is sweeter than a green one, and a black one is sweeter still.

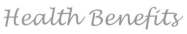

Health Benefits

- Helps relieve hemorrhoids
- Helps relieve skin reactions and inflammation insect bites, burns, etc.
- Helps relieve ulcers and inflammation in the mouth and pharynx
- Helps treat respiratory tract inflammation
- Lowers blood cholesterol levels

Put To Good Use

There is a definite health-giving benefit to replacing a side dish of potatoes or white pasta with plantain, a vegetable that harmonizes so well with meat dishes and fish.

Caution

Consumed in large amounts, plantain may have a laxative effect and may increase blood pressure.

Some people are allergic to plantain. If you have other food allergies, test a tiny amount to begin with.

Selecting & Storing

If a recipe calls for steamed plantain, choose fruits that are more yellow in ripeness, verging on black. For frying, choose fruit that are green. Plantain will keep for a little over a week at room temperature.

Culinary Use

It may be necessary to use a knife to separate the peel from the flesh of the plantain. It cooks like potato and can also be baked in the oven. Allow about one hour at 350ºF (180ºC). To take full advantage of the vegetable's healing properties, it is advisable to steam plantain rather than frying.

Recipe

- Plantains with Parsnip and Coriander (page 183)

Healthful Hints

To avoid discoloration of a plantain before cooking, plunge it into water containing a few drops of lemon juice.

To peel a plantain, slice the fruit length-wise, then remove the skin.

Good To Know

A type of fiber extracted from plantain is made into a powder that fortifies the cardiovascular system and also combats gastric ulcers.

Plum

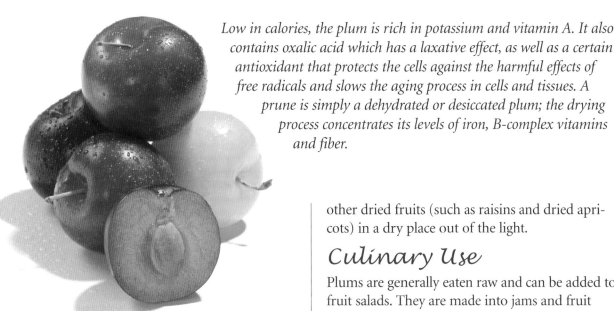

Low in calories, the plum is rich in potassium and vitamin A. It also contains oxalic acid which has a laxative effect, as well as a certain antioxidant that protects the cells against the harmful effects of free radicals and slows the aging process in cells and tissues. A prune is simply a dehydrated or desiccated plum; the drying process concentrates its levels of iron, B-complex vitamins and fiber.

Health Benefits

- Excellent source of energy
- Helps detoxify the liver
- Lowers levels of "bad" (LDL) cholesterol
- Relieves constipation

Home Remedy

Constipation remedy

Soak five or six prunes overnight and eat them first thing in the morning before breakfast. Drink the soaking water as well.

Caution

If taken in overly large quantities, prunes can cause flatulence, nausea and other gastric problems. To take full advantage of their healing properties, it is best to add them gradually and progressively to your diet.

Selecting & Storing

Choose plums that are firm with slight softness, with skins that are smooth and shiny. Store them in the refrigerator. Prunes should be stored like other dried fruits (such as raisins and dried apricots) in a dry place out of the light.

Culinary Use

Plums are generally eaten raw and can be added to fruit salads. They are made into jams and fruit sauces. Prunes can be added to rice, meat stews, desserts, crisps and squares, as well as 'stewed' mixtures of dried fruits.

Recipe

- Apple, Pear and Prune Purée (page 136)

Great Combinations

Add plums when cooking applesauce so as to boost the level of dietary fiber. This fruit sauce aids intestinal function and improves regularity. The pectin supplied by both fruits inhibits digestive tract irritations and helps restore efficient digestion.

Healthful Hints

You can replace refined sugar with prunes, dates or figs in many dessert recipes.

Good To Know

Commercially available prune juice, while lower in fiber, still possesses laxative properties.

P

Potato

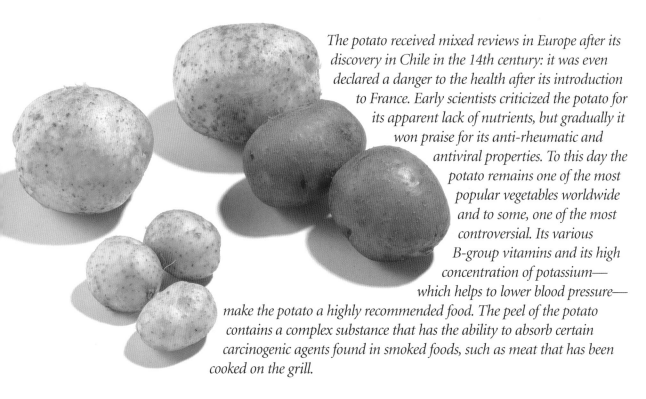

The potato received mixed reviews in Europe after its discovery in Chile in the 14th century: it was even declared a danger to the health after its introduction to France. Early scientists criticized the potato for its apparent lack of nutrients, but gradually it won praise for its anti-rheumatic and antiviral properties. To this day the potato remains one of the most popular vegetables worldwide and to some, one of the most controversial. Its various B-group vitamins and its high concentration of potassium— which helps to lower blood pressure— make the potato a highly recommended food. The peel of the potato contains a complex substance that has the ability to absorb certain carcinogenic agents found in smoked foods, such as meat that has been cooked on the grill.

Health Benefits

- Combats diabetes
- Helps in the treatment of skin diseases
- Helps prevent certain types of cancer
- Lowers blood pressure
- Relieves rheumatism

Put To Good Use

It is recommended that we eat the potato as a starch food for our evening meal (preferably with the peel) because of its relaxing effect that helps to bring on sleep.

It is, unfortunately, the raw, unpeeled potato that offers the most benefits for our health—a crunchy but not very tasty option! Baked potato with the skin on, is the next best thing since it retains most of the important heath-giving properties. Since they are low in calories, we can eat potatoes often, as long as we do not douse them with too much butter or sour cream.

Caution

Though specialists contradict each other on this point, the potato is not recommended for diabetics because of its high glycemic index. Wholegrain rice and oats are preferred sources of food energy.

Never cook or eat potatoes that have sprouted or have turned green. These should be discarded because they may have an increased level of solanin, a toxic substance found in the plants of the nightshade family.

Selecting & Storing

Different types of potato are good for different types of cooking: baked, French-fried, mashed or pan-fried. Popular varieties include Russet, Idaho and Yukon Gold. New potatoes—the small variety harvested in the summer—are good boiled and added to salads.

Choose potatoes without bruises or sprouts. They should be stored in a cool place—but not refrigerated—in a cloth or paper bag. Do not store potatoes with onions because an exchange of acids between these vegetables causes both to decompose more rapidly.

Culinary Use

Potatoes are prepared in a many appetizing ways, such as in salads, soups, vegetable side dishes, stews and baked vegetables *au gratin*.

Recipes

- Broccoli Soup (page 167)
- Cauliflower Soup (page 168)
- Curried Celery Soup (page 171)
- Mashed Potatoes with Carrot and Rutabaga (page 184)
- Parsnip and Zucchini Soup (page 169)
- Radish-Leaf Soup (page 172)

Great Combinations

To preserve the highest vitamin C content of potatoes, steam them with their skins on. Try steamed new potatoes sprinkled with fresh parsley and drizzled with olive oil. This combination is rich in vitamins B_9 and C, iron and beta carotene.

Healthful Hints

Good news for lovers of French fries: frozen French fries baked in the oven are considerably less fatty than those cooked in oil. The best way to make French fries is to toss unpeeled, coarsely-chopped potatoes in a bowl with 2 tbsp (60 ml) of grapeseed oil,

then arrange them on a cookie sheet and cook in a very hot oven for about 10 minutes. These homemade fries are a healthy alternative and are just as tasty as the deep-fried variety.

Good To Know

Despite what we might think about the starchy white color of potatoes, they do in fact supply a good source of antioxidants that protect us from a number of health conditions, notably cardiovascular disease. In some markets, potatoes are available in different colors (mauve, red and orange). These contain more than four times the level of antioxidants found in regular potatoes, giving them the capacity to neutralize free radicals in the body to an even greater degree than spinach or Brussels sprouts. Also note that the yellower the flesh of the potato, the greater the vitamin C content.

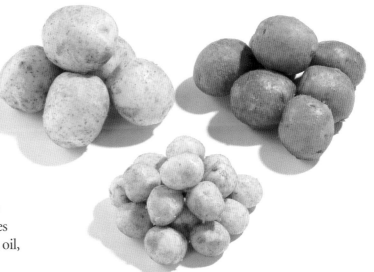

P

Quinoa

Originally cultivated in Peru, Ecuador and Bolivia, quinoa was the staple food of the Incas who called it the 'mother of all grains.' Technically not a cereal grain in the strict botanical sense, quinoa is a leafy plant from which the nutritious seeds are harvested. The seeds are very high in protein, containing all of the essential amino acids needed by the body—in particular the amino acids containing sulfur that are rarely found in plant proteins. Quinoa is also a good source of iron, magnesium, phosphorus and potassium, and contains almost all the B-group vitamins. Low in sodium, it also does not contain gluten.

Health Benefits

Quinoa combats fatigue and fortifies the body since the grain contains all eight essential amino acids. Research has shown that people who are weak due to an unhealthy diet regain their strength and boost their endurance after eating quinoa for just a few weeks.

Put To Good Use

People who are suffering from anemia, as well as celiacs (those suffering from gluten intolerance), will see a real improvement in their health if they include quinoa in their diet three or four times a week.

Caution

Quinoa seeds must always be washed several times before cooking so as to remove the residues of saponin, a natural waxy substance that the plant secretes on to the skin of the seed to protect itself from birds and insects.

Selecting & Storing

Quinoa is found at health food stores and in bulk food bins at some supermarkets. It is also sold as rolled flakes or flour.

Because of its high oil content, it is best to store quinoa in a sealed glass jar in a cool, dry place. Plan on using quinoa within a month of buying it.

Culinary Use

The delicate, light flavor of quinoa makes a tasty substitute for rice, bulgur or couscous in dishes like taboulé (page 216) or pilaf. Cook in twice its volume of water for about 10 minutes, until it curls inside out and appears translucent.

Quinoa is excellent for stuffings, stews and soups. One cup (250 ml) of raw quinoa cooked in a hot liquid (water, broth or vegetable juice) will yield three cups (750 ml) of cooked quinoa.

Recipes

- Chinese Cabbage Rolls (page 205)
- Couscous and Parsley Salad (Taboulé) (page 216)
- Corn and Quinoa Soup (page 174)

Great Combinations

Combine citrus fruits, parsley and quinoa. The acidity of lemon or orange and their vitamin C content is enriched by the iron of the parsley and will increase the fortifying and revitalizing effects of the quinoa.

Healthful Hints

Quinoa seeds can be browned in a saucepan for five minutes before cooking to give a grilled flavor.

Good To Know

According to historians, 10 million Incas at one time lived in the high plateaus of the Andes and survived thanks to the highly nutritious properties of quinoa. Because it is so rich in protein, quinoa offers the potential of solving the problem of hunger around the world.

Protein levels in quinoa (about 15 percent) are considerably higher than those of wheat (about 11.5 percent) and other grains. Quinoa also contains fewer carbohydrates than other grains.

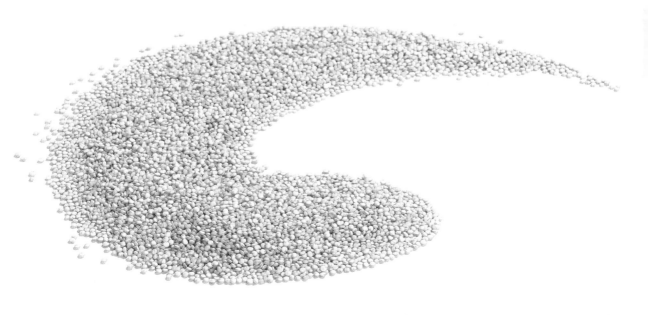

Q

Radish

This leafy garden plant, with its bright red, round peppery root, is in the cruciferae family, also called the mustard family (which includes the turnip, broccoli, cauliflower, Brussels sprout and cabbage). Like its cousins, the radish contains medicinal compounds that protect the body against certain forms of cancer. Rich in cellulose, vitamin C, potassium and iron, the radish is low in calories and possesses a number of preventive properties due to the sulfurous compounds it contains. For those who find the red radish difficult to digest, the black radish may be an alternative since it is renowned for aiding in digestion and stimulating the gall bladder. The black radish also has a reputation for treating respiratory infections.

Health Benefits

- Aids in digestion (black radish)
- Antiseptic
- Helps intestinal function
- Helps prevent cardiovascular disease
- Lowers the risk of cancer
- Soothes coughs (black radish)
- Stimulates appetite, fortifies the body

Home Remedy

Fortifying cough syrup

In a bowl, place alternating layers of black radish slices and coarse rock sugar that will melt very slowly. After about 12 hours, a syrup will have formed; take 4 to 6 tbsp (60 to 90 ml) a day to relieve a cough. This syrup is also an excellent fortifying tonic recommended for growing children.

Caution

People who are not used to eating red radishes should start out slowly and monitor their intake, avoid excessive consumption and eat only young, fresh roots.

The sulfurous compounds in the radish may inhibit the absorption of iodine by the body and cause problems with the proper functioning of the thyroid gland.

The black radish and its juice may be difficult for some people to digest. Those suffering from heartburn, indigestion, stomach ulcers or a thyroid illness should avoid it altogether.

It is not advisable to continue eating black radish for more than three consecutive weeks.

Selecting & Storing

Try to choose small radishes, since the larger ones often have hollow areas and tend to be less flavorful. Also note that round radishes tend to be sweeter than longer radishes. Pick radishes that are firm, without blemishes or bruises. Pay special attention to the leaves and be sure to pick only those that are healthy and green. Radishes will keep for about two weeks in the vegetable drawer of the refrigerator.

Culinary Use

Both red and black radishes are eaten raw in salads and appetizers, although the black radish will also retain its healthy properties in soups.

The daikon, or white radish, is usually grated before serving, and can be served marinated in soy sauce or tamari. The Japanese are very fond of daikon radish as an hors d'oeuvre, sprinkled with rice vinegar, used with dips or as a side dish for fish, sea food or chicken, or as a garnish for sushi and sashimi. They also enjoy the leaves of the radish, as well as the sprouted seeds.

Recipe

- Radish-Leaf Soup (page 172)

Great Combinations

Raw red radish, cut in oval slices or short sticks and added to mixed salads, will enrich the vitamin C content of those vegetables lacking the vitamin, such as tomatoes, carrots and cucumber.

Healthful Hints

Radish leaves are rich in vitamins and should not be forgotten. They are quite delicious in soups (see page 172).

To make radish sprouts, soak seeds for 8 to 14 hours before placing in a glass jar. Then follow the same sprouting technique used for sprouting flaxseed (page 56). Young, day-old radish sprouts can be eaten or they can be left to grow for a further two or three days. Only small quantities of radish sprouts should be added to salads and sandwiches: they are noticeably spicy!

Good To Know

A black radish contains more vitamin C than an orange. It is one of the best sources of vitamin C because it is almost always eaten raw, whereas other vegetables will lose a significant amount of their vitamin content through cooking.

Raspberry

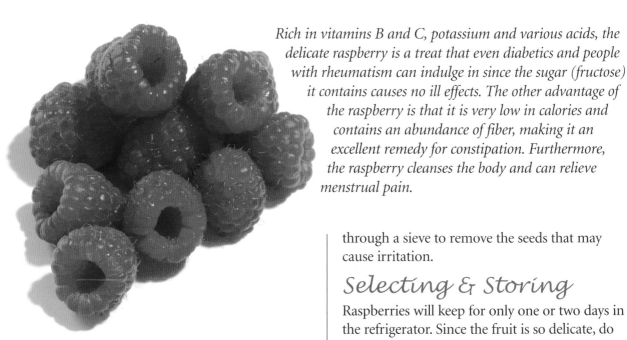

Rich in vitamins B and C, potassium and various acids, the delicate raspberry is a treat that even diabetics and people with rheumatism can indulge in since the sugar (fructose) it contains causes no ill effects. The other advantage of the raspberry is that it is very low in calories and contains an abundance of fiber, making it an excellent remedy for constipation. Furthermore, the raspberry cleanses the body and can relieve menstrual pain.

Health Benefits

- Anti-rheumatic
- Cleansing and detoxifying
- Combats mouth sores and inflammation
- Combats urinary tract infections
- Diuretic
- Helps protect cells from aging
- Increases intestinal digestion
- Lowers the risk of cardiovascular disease
- Soothes upset stomach and indigestion

Put To Good Use

Added to breakfast cereals, raspberries are an excellent source of dietary fiber, which, we now know, plays an important role in protecting the body from cardiovascular disease.

Caution

People who have a sensitive intestinal tract or Irritable Bowel Syndrome (IBS) are advised to eat strained raspberries; here, the fruit is passed through a sieve to remove the seeds that may cause irritation.

Selecting & Storing

Raspberries will keep for only one or two days in the refrigerator. Since the fruit is so delicate, do not wash until just before eating.

Culinary Use

Served raw, raspberries are an excellent, refreshing snack that, topped with yogurt, becomes a truly exquisite delicacy.

Recipe

- Fruit Cup with Mango Cream (page 234)

Healthful Hints

Pectinase, the natural enzyme that breaks down the pectin in raspberries, starts acting fairly soon after the berries are picked and makes it more difficult to turn them into jelly. For this reason, it is important to obtain the freshest, most recently picked raspberries for making jams and jellies.

Good To Know

Raspberry leaves have astringent, diuretic and laxative properties. An old English recipe of raspberry leaves made an herb tea that was given to pregnant women during childbirth.

Rice

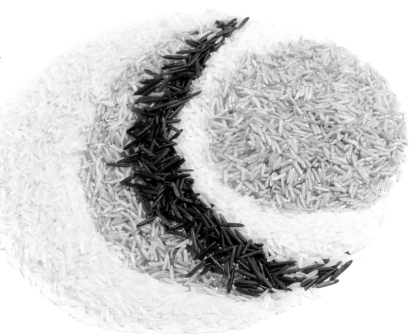

Along with wheat, rice is the most widely consumed grain on earth. Of the 8,000 or so varieties available on five continents, it is wholegrain brown rice, with its long brown kernel, that is the most nutritious. Highly digestible, it is rich in minerals and soluble dietary fiber—the kind of fiber known to lower the risk of heart disease and protect against various forms of cancer.

Health Benefits

- Combats diarrhea
- Lowers blood pressure
- Lowers levels of blood cholesterol
- Reduces the risk of cardiovascular disease
- Reduces the risk of colon, breast and prostate cancer
- Relieves kidney afflictions

Home Remedy

Relief from diarrhea

For centuries mothers have made their children drink a thin porridge of rice to combat diarrhea. Simply boil ½ cup (125 ml) of well-rinsed brown rice in 4 cups (1 liter) of salted water for 10 minutes.

Put To Good Use

There are definite health benefits to eating brown rice several times a week, thanks to the preventive properties of wholegrain rice.

Because rice contains no gluten, it can be safely eaten by people with celiac disease.

Caution

Regular white rice, which undergoes several stages of cleaning and processing, is stripped of much of its dietary fiber and many of its health-giving properties. However, thiamin and niacin are added to white rice, making it a rich source of vitamin B_3.

Selecting & Storing

You will find all sorts of rice available at the supermarket: short-grain rice for sushi and puddings; Arborio rice for risottos; long-grain rice such as wehani; and perfumed rice like basmati, Thai or jasmine rice. Despite the choices, it is still wholegrain rice—either red, brown or black (wild rice)—that has been proven to be the most nutritious. Since wholegrain rice will spoil faster than white rice, it should be stored in a sealed container in the refrigerator, where it will keep for up to a year.

Culinary Use

Rice is an essential staple food, especially in Southern Asia where it is indispensable and is

R

present in any proper meal. In other parts of the world, it is readily used as a side dish, for soups and even for desserts.

Short- and medium-grain rice are known for being richer in starch, and they have a tendency to be stickier once cooked. They are mainly used in sushi, dumplings, meats stuffed with rice, soups and desserts.

Long-grain rice contains a different kind of starch that keeps the grains separate when cooked. Apart from being the main rice of India (basmati) and China (jasmine), it is the most popular type of rice in the West and is used in a wide variety of dishes.

Recipes

- Brown Rice with Almond and Raisin (page 185)
- Chinese Cabbage Rolls (page 205)
- Curried Rice with Pistachio (page 184)
- Indian-Style Rice and Sweet Potato Pie (page 186)
- Lentil Curry with Pistachio (page 193)
- Rice with Leek, Mushroom and Fine Herbs (page 185)

Healthful Hints

Rice can be flavored in any number of ways since a variety of food ingredients can be added to it, each lending their own unique flavors. Consider adding vegetables or dried fruits to rice before cooking, or pulses (like chickpeas and lentils), nuts and spices, cheese, meat, fish or shellfish.

Good To Know

Wild rice is an aquatic plant harvested by North American native peoples and belongs to a completely different genus from regular rice. Very high in protein, wild rice contains the eight essential amino acids, making it quite similar to oats in its nutritional content. The very long, dark grains of wild rice must be cooked longer than ordinary brown rice—for up to a whole hour.

Long-grain brown rice, or wholegrain rice, has a pleasing nutty flavor and undergoes only a basic polishing process to remove the husk, leaving its layers of bran untouched. This bran contains many of the vitamins, minerals and fiber—health-giving nutrients that are removed from regular white or parboiled rice.

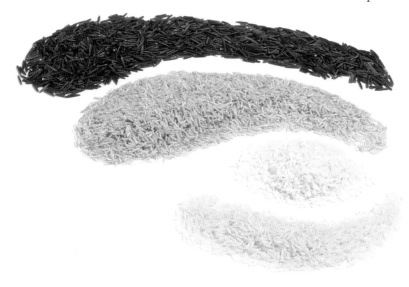

Rye

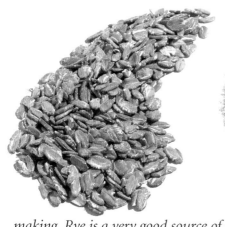 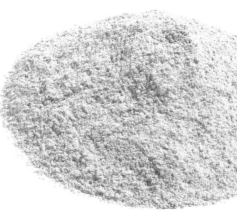

Very popular in Eastern Europe, Scandinavia and Russia (all countries where the incidence of cardiovascular disease and atherosclerosis is low), rye is used almost exclusively for bread making. Rye is a very good source of vitamin E, the B-group vitamins, minerals and it also contains rutin, an antioxidant compound that strengthens the blood vessels and promotes circulation. Rye is especially recommended for sedentary people or those who are bed-ridden or wheelchair-bound.

Health Benefits

- Helps prevent atherosclerosis (hardening of the arteries)
- Lowers blood pressure
- Protects against cardiovascular disease

Put To Good Use

Delicious when toasted, rye bread is even better than whole wheat bread at breakfast time and should be alternated with whole wheat bread. Regular consumption of rye bread also keeps the skin healthy and fresh, and can help in slowing the development of wrinkles.

Caution

As with wheat, oats and barley, rye contains a number of proteins, including gliadins that cause an allergic reaction in celiacs (those allergic to gluten).

Selecting & Storing

Rye has a texture similar to wheat but its color is darker and its flavor is more pronounced. The grain is sold whole, rolled or milled into flour. It is stored like other cereal grains, in a sealed container in a cool, dry place out of the direct light.

Culinary Use

Rye cooks like most other grains, taking between 60 and 90 minutes; it doubles its size in water.

Recipe

- Homemade Granola (page 139)

Healthful Hints

Rye bread is great when used for sandwiches or as an extra-healthy bun for a hamburger, garnished with slices of onion, tomato and goat's cheese.

Good To Know

In some regions, rye grain is being phased out completely and replaced with a cross of wheat and rye called triticale. The two grains are also being grown in combination.

R

Seaweed

For centuries, seaweeds have been eaten in the Far East, notably Japan, and in some areas of maritime Europe and North America. Only recently has it become more widespread in North America, due to our growing interest in Asian cuisine. Now, health-conscious gourmet chefs are including seaweed in their creations. These fresh and saltwater algae contain a wealth of vitamins, minerals and dietary fiber, as well as compounds with proven antibiotic properties. Often found in the pharmaceutical industry, seaweeds such as spirulina and bladder wrack are sold as dietary supplements.

Health Benefits

- Anti-rheumatic and antibiotic
- Fortifying tonic
- Helps treat anemia
- Lowers both cholesterol and blood sugar levels
- Slows the growth of tumors

Put To Good Use

Since seaweeds are rich in sea salt, add crumbled seaweed to an unsalted broth as a salt substitute to boost its vitamin and mineral content.

Caution

Consume in moderation: over-consumption of seaweed can cause skin problems, an overloading of minerals and irregularities of the thyroid gland.

Do not over-rinse seaweed since its health-giving properties may be washed away.

Selecting & Storing

Seaweeds in health food stores are generally dried and can be easily stored for months in a sealed bag or container.

Culinary Use

Wakame, which looks like a large serrated leaf, is used in soups, sauces and salads, and makes a good accompaniment to rice and tofu.

Thongweed, or sea spaghetti, is a long fine, green seaweed that goes well with fish. Dulse, a red seaweed found in the northern Atlantic and Pacific regions, is eaten raw, dried or used as a food flavor enhancer.

Recipes

- Carrots and Parsnips with Dulse (page 151)
- Onion Soup with Dulse (page 172)

Healthful Hints

To get all the health-giving properties out of seaweed, use them in soups so that the nutrients will be released into the broth.

Another excellent, convenient way to include seaweed in your diet is to sprinkle tiny flakes like a seasoning onto cooked vegetables, soups and main course dishes with sauce.

Good To Know

Recent studies have shown that a type of blue-green algae, spirulina, contains almost twice as much protein as soy flour (weight for weight). For centuries, spirulina was made into cakes by the Aztecs and some tribes in Chad. Today it is available as a dietary supplement.

Soybean

The seed of this Asian plant from the legume family has been cultivated for several millennia by the Chinese, who refer to it as 'meat from the earth.' Recent studies in the West have uncovered an amazing number of health-giving properties found in the miraculous soybean. Most nations of the world are now integrating this legume into their food supply. It has been found that tofu and tempeh (two forms of fermented soybean) and soy 'milk' drinks have powerful therapeutic properties in addition to being rich in protein, vitamins and minerals. And since clinical research into the health benefits of soybeans and soy food products is still in its infancy, the potential exists for yet more discoveries that will have positive effects on the health of men, women and children around the globe.

Health Benefits

- Helps intestinal function
- Helps prevent cardiovascular disease
- Helps stabilize blood sugar levels
- Lowers levels of "bad" (LDL) cholesterol
- Lowers the risk of breast, prostate and colon cancer
- Relieves symptoms related to menopause

Home Remedy

Battling "bad" (LDL) cholesterol

To reduce levels of LDL cholesterol, we are recommended to eat about 1 oz (30 g) of soy protein each day. Be careful to choose soy products low in unsaturated fat (less than 3 g), saturated fat (less than 1 g) and cholesterol (less than 20 mg), and without added fat.

Put To Good Use

Recent studies are suggesting that eating just one serving of a soy-based food dealy is sufficient to help reduce the risk of cancer.

Caution

Fermented soy products are not recommended for people who are sensitive to the effects of mold and mildew. The number of adults allergic to soybean products has increased considerably in recent years—no doubt due to the increased use of soy-based products in the food industry.

Tofu is a good source of calcium as long as the coagulant used in its composition is either calcium chloride or calcium sulfate. Read the label carefully to ensure that one of these ingredients is indeed present.

Selecting & Storing

There are dozens of soy-based food products: meat substitutes in the form of soy burgers or sausages, soy flour, flavored soy beverages, tempeh (a whole bean tofu), textured soy protein, and tofu—without a doubt the most popular form due to its ease of use in cooking. Tofu is a kind of cheese made from the soybean 'milk' and is available in either soft or firm blocks. Once the package has been opened, tofu will keep for about five days

S

in the refrigerator, in water that must be changed daily.

Culinary Use

It is said that tofu is something of a chameleon food in the sense that it takes on the flavors of whatever it is cooked with, as if to hide its relative tastelessness. It is preferable, therefore, to let tofu marinate (see below) before using. To take full advantage of its health-giving properties, we recommend not overcooking, and adding tofu only during the last few minutes of cooking. Tofu is included in a wide variety of dishes ranging from soups and salads to desserts.

Recipes

- Orange and Cherry Soy Smoothie (page 135)
- Quiche with Millet, Tofu and Lentils (page 203)
- Soy Milk with Mango (page 139)
- Spaghetti with Meatless Bolognaise Sauce (page 206)
- Tofu Burgers (page 191)
- Tofu Chili (page 197)
- Tofu Mayonnaise (page 224)

Healthful Hints

People who are interested in lowering their meat consumption can do so by gradually replacing their animal protein with diced tofu in pasta sauces and stews. This healthy change will allow you to explore and experiment with a whole new range of recipes.

A marinade for tofu or tempeh

Combine three equal parts of olive oil, apple cider vinegar and tamari, add a large clove of minced garlic, 1 tsp (5 ml) of grated fresh ginger, 1 tsp (5 ml) of curry powder and a few flakes of chili pepper. Add a block of tofu or tempeh and leave the mixture to marinate for two hours before adding to a stir-fry or stew. Do not cook it for longer than 10 minutes.

Good To Know

In terms of protein content, soy is the only plant source that can compare with meat, fish and eggs. When soy products and whole grains are eaten together, you can be assured of achieving the full complement of proteins that the body needs—the formula for a successful vegetarian diet.

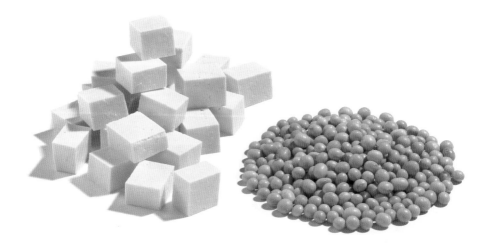

Spinach

The crisp, green leaves of spinach make for a very rich source of dietary fiber, vitamins C and E, chlorophyll and minerals. But it is the high content of carotenoids (including beta carotene) that makes spinach the cancer-fighting vegetable par excellence—on a par with cabbage. Studies have shown that people who regularly consume spinach are generally at a lower risk of developing a wide variety of cancers, including lung cancer.
For many dieticians, spinach has also usurped green beans as the best weight-loss food.

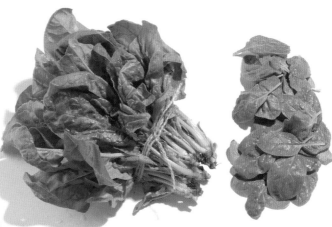

Health Benefits

- Combats depression
- Fortifies the heart, combats anemia
- Helps maintain good eyesight
- Helps regulate intestinal function
- Lowers levels of blood cholesterol
- Protects against different types of cancer
- Stimulates the pancreas, promotes insulin production

Put To Good Use

Eat fresh spinach raw with other leafy vegetables (see Lettuce) at least twice a week as an unbeatable preventive for many illnesses, and a regulator of mood and temperament.

Caution

For certain individuals with urinary tract problems, spinach may further aggravate the condition or promote the formation of kidney stones.

The high content of oxalic acid in spinach has a negative effect on calcium absorption, thus it should be consumed in moderation by people with any kind of calcium deficiency.

Selecting & Storing

Choose crisp, healthy green leaves—preferably those that are younger and smaller. Spinach leaves will keep for five to six weeks in the refrigerator in a perforated plastic bag.

Culinary Use

Raw, mixed with other salad greens, spinach makes excellent, highly nutritious salads.

Cooked, spinach makes a tasty vegetable side dish and goes well in soups, stews, vegetables baked *au gratin* or in filo pastry. It is also a delicious, colorful garnish for meat dishes.

Recipes

- Cabbage Salad with Clementine, Spinach and Sesame (page 215)
- Spinach and Mushroom Lasagna (page 200)
- Spinach and Tomato *au Gratin* (page 152)
- Spinach Soup with Pecans (page 170)
- Vegetable Pasta Salad with Feta (page 217)

Healthful Hints

Add a pinch of nutmeg to the cooking water of spinach to give a delicate, pleasing flavor.

Bon à savoir

It has been discovered recently that spinach—for decades hailed as an excellent source of iron—in fact contains 10 times less iron than originally thought. Its reputation as a health food was based on a simple mathematical error. In determining the iron content, a scientist misplaced a decimal—but it was a healthy mistake!

S

Squash

The winter squashes, harvested in late summer, include four main varieties: the caramel-colored, bell-shaped butternut squash; the gnarly, green and orange Hubbard squash; the neatly ridged, deep-green acorn squash; and the yellow, oval-shaped spaghetti squash. (For summer squash, see Zucchini.) In a single serving, the butternut and Hubbard each offer more than the daily recommended amount of carotene. All squashes are high in vitamin C and are an excellent source of dietary fiber.

Health Benefits

- Helps in preventing cardiovascular diseases
- Helps in preventing pulmonary afflictions
- Lowers the risk of uterine cancer
- Relieves constipation
- Relieves hemorrhoids

Put To Good Use

Asthma sufferers would benefit from eating winter squash regularly because of its high vitamin C content.

Caution

As far as it is known, there are no negative side-effects or allergies associated with squash.

Selecting & Storing

Choose squash that are heavy with thick skins; this will allow them to store for several weeks—possibly the whole winter—in a cool, dry place (at about 53ºF, or 12ºC). Choose a squash that still has its stem (peduncle); this reduces the likelihood of the flesh inside rotting.

Culinary Use

Combine butternut squash with carrots and rutabagas (yellow turnip) to make a delicious purée. Acorn squash (either green or white varieties) is very flavorful when cut in half, stuffed with a rice or meat mixture and baked in the oven. Hubbard squash is delicious cut into pie-shaped wedges and baked, or else peeled and cubed in stews to provide extra vitamins.

Recipe

- Butternut Squash Soup (page 167)

Healthful Hints

The thick, tough skin of the squash, which Mother Nature devised to protect its delicate inner flesh, is often quite difficult to remove. To make the job easier, start by cooking the whole squash in the oven before trying to slice it. After 20 minutes at 375ºF (190ºC), the skin should have softened, making slicing and peeling much easier.

Good To Know

The darker the orange of the squash's flesh, the higher the beta carotene content (that remarkable antioxidant that protects against cardiovascular afflictions).

Strawberry

Rich in vitamins and minerals, this small, delicious fruit can be eaten by diabetics because the form of sugar it contains (fructose) does not cause problems with blood sugar levels. Along with cantaloupe and raspberry, the strawberry is one of the three best weight-loss fruits. Strawberries also contain glutathion, an antioxidant that, according to recent studies, has the effect of slowing the deterioration of the immune system in people infected with HIV. Furthermore, the strawberry shares the top of the podium with the kiwi for fruits that have the highest concentration of vitamin C, another extremely important antioxidant.

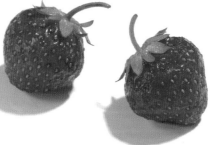

Health Benefits

- Diuretic and detoxifies
- Helps combat HIV
- Helps prevent constipation
- Relieves gout

Put To Good Use

It is recommended that we eat a few fresh strawberries each day as an appetizer before a meal.

Caution

Strawberries are not recommended for people with dermatitis. They may cause an allergic reaction or skin rash (but this usually disappears after eating the fruit). People who get an itching sensation on the lips from eating strawberries may have Oral Allergy Syndrome (see page 86).

Selecting & Storing

Avoid strawberries with white, unripe portions since they will not ripen further. Eat them as soon as possible after picking. They will keep for only two or three days in the refrigerator. To freeze, arrange fruit on a cookie sheet and transfer to sealed freezer bags once they are frozen.

Culinary Use

Strawberries make delicious jams, as well as garnishes for cakes and pies. Fresh, they add a refreshing burst of flavor to a salad.

Recipes

- Cranberry-Strawberry Purée (page 234)
- Strawberry... Avocado Salad (page 157)

Beauty Secret

Strawberry mask

Before bed, crush a few strawberries and spread on the face for at least an hour. (If possible, leave on overnight and rinse clean in the morning.) The mask brightens the complexion, relaxes lines and diminishes wrinkles.

Healthful Hints

Soak strawberries in red wine for an hour to sterilize. They can then be served as a delicious appetizer, sprinkled with a little sugar.

Good To Know

A 3-oz (100-g) portion of strawberries contains almost the full daily amount of vitamin C recommended by nutritionists.

Sweet Potato

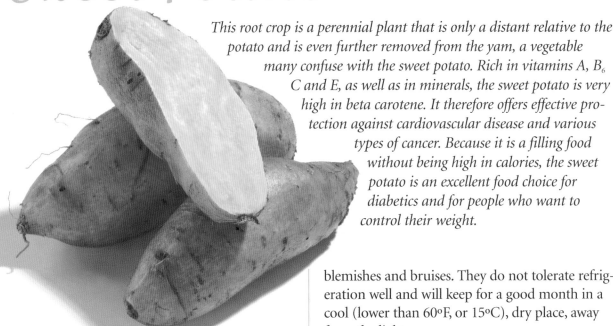

This root crop is a perennial plant that is only a distant relative to the potato and is even further removed from the yam, a vegetable many confuse with the sweet potato. Rich in vitamins A, B$_6$ C and E, as well as in minerals, the sweet potato is very high in beta carotene. It therefore offers effective protection against cardiovascular disease and various types of cancer. Because it is a filling food without being high in calories, the sweet potato is an excellent food choice for diabetics and for people who want to control their weight.

Health Benefits

- Cleanses and detoxifies
- Helps mental function and improves memory
- Lowers blood sugar levels
- Lowers the risk of cancer

Put To Good Use

Because of its many benefits, the sweet potato is healthier than the potato as an accompaniment to fish and meat dishes.

Caution

Beta carotene requires some fat in order to be absorbed by the small intestine, so be sure to eat some animal or vegetable fats alongside the sweet potato to maximize its healing properties.

Selecting & Storing

Choose roots with a rich orange color. As with all fruits and vegetables containing beta carotene, the orange-yellow color should be strong and bright. Sweet potatoes should be firm, smooth and free of blemishes and bruises. They do not tolerate refrigeration well and will keep for a good month in a cool (lower than 60ºF, or 15ºC), dry place, away from the light.

Culinary Use

Sweet potato cooks like regular potato: boiled, fried, mashed, added to salads, soups or stews. Because of its sweetness, it is also used in cakes and desserts.

Recipes

- Indian-Style Rice and Sweet Potato Pie (page 186)
- Sweet Potato and Celeriac Soup (page 171)
- Vegetable Chick-Pea Casserole *au Gratin* (page 196)

Healthful Hints

From amongst the varieties of creamy or orange sweet potatoes, choose those with a lovely, bright orange color to ensure a high level of beta carotene.

Good To Know

A 4-oz (120-g) portion of sweet potato contains 28 mg of vitamin C: roughly half the recommended daily allowance.

Tea

Although tea is now the most popular drink on the planet, the therapeutic properties of its dried leaves were already known over 4,000 years ago in China. In addition to stimulating digestion, tea has recently been the focus of scientific studies examining its antioxidant properties, which are believed to inhibit the development of cancer and combat cardiovascular disease. Without added sugar or milk, tea is a beverage that is very low in both calories and sodium.

Health Benefits

- Combats atherosclerosis (hardening of the arteries)
- Helps destroy viruses and bacteria
- Helps prevent cavities and gum disease
- Helps relieve diarrhea
- Lowers blood pressure
- Lowers the risk of cancer
- Sharpens the mental capacities
- Stimulates digestion

Put To Good Use

A cup of tea between meals is a healthy replacement for a cup of coffee, from the point of view of its therapeutic properties. However, since tea also contains caffeine, it is recommended that not more than three cups be consumed per day.

Caution

The tannins found in tea may cause a slowing of the body's absorption of minerals (such as iron). This can be countered by drinking tea only between meals, or else by adding iron-rich foods to your diet.

Regular, frequent tea drinking may cause brown stains on the teeth.

It is not recommended that women drink tea (or coffee) during pregnancy, since theine, the form of caffeine found in tea, may have adverse effects.

Nursing mothers should drink tea in moderate amounts since the theine may be transmitted to the infant through breast milk, causing sleeplessness.

Tea should not be given to infants or children, since they may have adverse reactions to the tannins and theine.

T

Selecting & Storing

Among the most common types of tea, of special note are black tea (including Darjeeling and English breakfast); oolong tea, made from green tea leaves partly heated and dried; and green tea, with a more bitter yet more thirst-quenching flavor. Dried tea keeps easily in a sealed opaque container and should never be refrigerated since the cold and humidity will cause it to lose its flavors.

Culinary Use

An ideal digestive drink, a cup of tea puts the finishing touches on an excellent meal.

Recipe

- Green Tea with Ginger and Mint (page 246)

Healthful Hints

Decaffeinated tea

A portion of the caffeine (theine) of tea can be removed by discarding the first infusion of the leaves after steeping for one minute. Theine diffuses rapidly from the leaves into the hot water.

Beauty Secret

Tea bags for baggy eyes

To help get rid of bags under the eyes and to relax muscles, placed cooled, still-humid tea bags on the eyelids for a few minutes.

Good To Know

Tea is rich in antioxidant compounds called flavonoids that have an important effect throughout the body. According to recent studies, a cup of tea will provide the same number of health benefits as a glass of red wine, without the side effects. Flavonoids also combat cancer (of both the esophagus and the skin).

Moreover, bone health appears to be superior among people who have regularly consumed tea for over 10 years. The consumption of tea also seems to stimulate the action of insulin in diabetics, having a favorable effect on their blood sugar levels.

Contrary to popular belief, however, tea does not help weight loss. On the other hand, a cup of tea contains virtually no calories, as long as you don't add milk or sugar. It is therefore a drink that will not cause any gain in weight.

Tea in bags contains the same number of antioxidants as tea leaves. To take full advantage of the health-giving properties of tea, leaves or bags should be infused in freshly boiled water for a full three minutes.

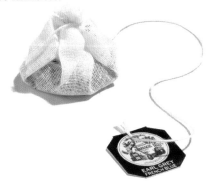

Tomato

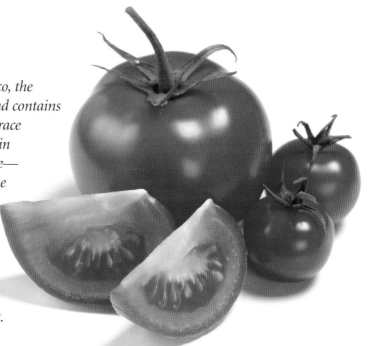

The fruit of a plant originally from Mexico, the tomato is rich in vitamins A, B and C, and contains an abundance of essential minerals and trace elements. Low in calories, tomatoes contain lycopene—a close relative of beta carotene— which accounts for its bright red color. The antioxidant properties of lycopene have been shown to be particularly effective in helping to both prevent and combat prostate cancer. Contrary to the popular belief that tomatoes are acidic, they are in fact alkaline and present no danger to people with arthritis, rheumatism or gout.

Health Benefits

- Helps in the digestion of starches
- Helps in the prevention of appendicitis
- Helps prevent cataracts
- Lowers the risk of certain types of cancer (breast, digestive tract, prostate, lung, uterine)

Put To Good Use

Consumed daily, raw tomatoes in salads or cooked tomatoes in sauces and soups reduce the harmful effects of free radicals and, according to published reports, can help prevent various types of cancer. Reliable evidence shows that people who consume tomatoes seven times a week, no matter what the format, are only half as likely to develop cancer as people who eat them less often.

Caution

When consumed in large amounts, tomatoes may cause an allergic reaction and negatively affect the stomachs of people who suffer from heartburn and indigestion.

Green tomatoes should be avoided as they are known to cause migraine headaches. Under-ripe tomatoes will ripen faster if wrapped in newspaper and left at room temperature for a few days.

People who are allergic to aspirin should not eat tomatoes.

Selecting & Storing

Color is often the best criterion when choosing tomatoes. A fully ripe tomato with a rich red color tastes the best, and indeed is the best for you since it contains four times the beta carotene of green tomatoes. Tomatoes do not need to be kept in the refrigerator; they keep perfectly for a couple of days at room temperature.

Culinary Use

One of the most versatile fresh 'fruits,' the tomato can be used in anything from appetizers and drinks to desserts, and it adapts well to any number of sauces. It is an essential ingredient that lends its rich and energizing flavor to a variety of hot and cold dishes.

T

Recipes

- Braised Fennel in Tomato Sauce (page 181)
- Fresh Tomato Sauce (microwave recipe) (page 226)
- Pasta Puttanesca (page 202)
- Ratatouille Niçoise (page 155)
- Spaghetti with Eggplant and Shiitake Mushrooms (page 207)
- Spinach and Mushroom Lasagna (page 200)
- Spinach and Tomato *au Gratin* (page 152)
- Tagliatelle with Lentil Sauce (page 208)
- Tomato Salad with Fresh Basil (page 158)
- Vegetable Pasta Salad with Feta (page 217)
- Walnut-Stuffed Tomatoes (page 159)

Healthful Hint

Peeling and seeding fresh tomatoes

It is best to peel tomatoes before cooking. To do this easily, cut a cross into the bottom of the tomato, drop it into boiling water for about one minute, then drop into a bowl of iced water. After a short time—the time it takes to cool—the skin should be easy to remove.

To remove seeds, cut the tomato horizontally and pull out the seeds while pressing gently on the edges.

Dried tomatoes

Make your own dried tomatoes by cutting Italian tomatoes in half (if small) or in slices, and spread them on a baking sheet. Cook at 200ºF (100ºC) until dry (roughly 6 to 12 hours). Store in a sealed container in the refrigerator.

Beauty Secret

Healthy skin, fresh complexion

To cleanse the skin of impurities, nothing can beat a tomato mask. Simply peel a tomato and remove the seeds. Crush with a fork and apply to the face for fifteen minutes. Rinse with lukewarm water.

Healthful Hints

Tomato leaves for insect bites

Fresh, crumpled tomato leaves rubbed on insect bites will help relieve the itching.

Good To Know

Cooking preserves the health-giving nutrients of the tomato and helps to release the antioxidant lycopene, an effective cancer-fighting agent.

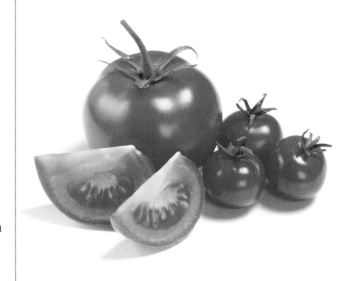

Turmeric

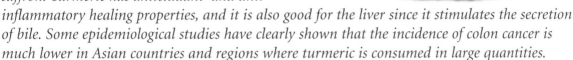

Known and used for a few millennia in traditional Indian Ayurvedic medicine, turmeric is a spice that is rich in vitamin C, iron and potassium. It is often called the "saffron of India" due to the strong yellow-colored pigment called curcumin found in the root of the plant. But the similarities end there because its somewhat bitter taste is far spicier than saffron. Turmeric has antioxidant and anti-inflammatory healing properties, and it is also good for the liver since it stimulates the secretion of bile. Some epidemiological studies have clearly shown that the incidence of colon cancer is much lower in Asian countries and regions where turmeric is consumed in large quantities.

Health Benefits

- Aids digestion
- Antiseptic and anti-spasmodic
- Combats joint inflammation, arthrosis and arthritis
- Helps prevent Alzheimer's disease
- Helps prevent cataracts
- Helps to heal skin afflictions
- Lowers the risk of cancer, notably skin cancer
- Relieves arthritic pain
- Relieves diarrhea, combats intestinal parasites

Home Remedies

For digestive problems

Infuse about 1 tsp (5 ml) turmeric in ⅔ cup (150 ml) of boiling water for 10 to 15 minutes. Drink two glasses a day.

Also, ¾ tsp (4 ml) of turmeric three times per week, sprinkled in soups, vegetable dishes, or sauces, offers excellent protection against infections of all kinds.

Caution

Sufferers of gastric (stomach) ulcers should avoid turmeric since a study has revealed that the curcumin compound, in higher doses, may be an irritant to the stomach.

Selecting & Storing

It is best to buy turmeric in small quantities as its medicinal properties will deteriorate over time.

Culinary Use

The spice, which is also used as a dye in India, is a key ingredient in the preparation of many curries (masala), and it gives color and an exotic aroma to soups, rice dishes and meat stews.

Recipes

- Curried Rice with Pistachio (page 184)
- Indian-Style Braised Cauliflower (page 179)
- Lentil Curry with Pistachio (page 193)
- Quiche with Millet, Tofu and Lentils (page 203)

Beauty Secret

In India, a paste of turmeric is applied to the face as a ceremonial beauty mask.

Good To Know

The darker the turmeric powder, the better the quality.

T

Turnip

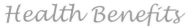

Even though the turnip contains few minerals and only minor amounts of potassium, sulfur, calcium and vitamin C, it has proven to be rich in compounds that inhibit the progress of cancer in laboratory animals. As with other members of the mustard family (cabbage, broccoli, radish, and its close cousin the rutabaga), the turnip, with its yellow flesh, contains several cancer-fighting compounds. Both turnip and rutabaga are recommended for people who are trying to lose weight.

Health Benefits

- Helps intestinal function
- Low in calories
- Lowers the risk of colon and rectal cancers

Put To Good Use

Eaten raw twice a week like carrot sticks, turnip and rutabaga offer protection again cancer.

Caution

The sulfur contained in turnips may slow digestion and cause flatulence.

Selecting & Storing

Choose a turnip root that is firm, smooth and heavy, without wrinkles, blemishes or bruises. Turnip leaves have a slightly sweet flavor and can be cooked like spinach. The leaves contain beta carotene and vitamin C.

Culinary Use

Turnip and rutabaga cook like carrots and give a delicious, hearty flavor to soups, puréed vegetables and stews. However, if you want to take full advantage of all the health-giving properties of the turnip, you should eat it raw.

Recipes

- Mashed Potatoes with Carrot and Rutabaga (page 184)
- Vegetable Chick-Pea Casserole *au Gratin* (page 196)

A Perfect Combination

Garnish a roasted duck or leg of lamb with cooked turnip. The low-calorie turnip helps to lighten and balance out the richness of the meat fats and contributes dietary fiber and minerals such as potassium, calcium and sulfur. Do not add oil or other fats while roasting the meat: simply keep it moist with a broth or white wine.

Healthful Hints

Try grating turnip and adding it to a little clarified butter in a saucepan. Cooked in this simple, delicious and healthy manner, turnips become a great side dish for roast beef or grilled salmon.

Good To Know

Turnip is more digestible when not overcooked.

Walnut

The Persian walnut is the most commonly available variety and is often called the English walnut, dating from a time when the British controlled much of the world's walnut trade. Rich in minerals, vitamin E and some B vitamins, fresh, unroasted walnuts also contain vitamin C. The walnut is an oily nut and is therefore high in calories, but it contains several other compounds including omega-3 fatty acids that help to prevent cardiovascular disease.

Health Benefits

- Helps prevent cardiovascular disease
- Helps treat diarrhea and is a laxative
- Lowers cholesterol levels
- Protects against cancer

Put To Good Use

If you foresee a physically demanding day ahead requiring more effort than usual, try blending one glass of fruit juice of your choice with a handful of walnuts as a fortifying tonic. Do not over-indulge in this delicious, high-energy drink, and do not drink it every day, especially if you are trying to lose weight.

Caution

As with all nuts, walnuts can provoke serious allergic reactions in certain people.

Also, because walnuts are very high in fats, they should be consumed in small quantities only, especially if they are being added progressively to your diet to replace another high-calorie food.

Selecting & Storing

Walnuts can be bought whole (unshelled), shelled, chopped or ground. It is preferable to buy nuts in shops with a high turnover of produce since they will go rancid after a few weeks. Choose nuts that feel heavy for their size and store them in a sealed container in a cool place out of the light. Whole walnuts freeze well and do not need to be thawed before using.

Culinary Use

Walnuts add their bittersweet flavor to sautéed vegetables or salads, transforming an everyday dish into something quite sophisticated. They also play a part in many delicious desserts and add flavor and richness to dishes containing tofu and grains.

Recipes

- Almond (or Walnut) Butter (page 247)
- Mushroom and Walnut Spread (page 154)
- Walnut-Stuffed Tomatoes (page 159)

A Perfect Combination

Add walnuts to your bread or muffin recipes. The nuts will boost the mineral content of the bread, notably calcium, iron, magnesium, sulfur and zinc—nutrients that are usually absent from bread.

Healthful Hints

Try making your own delicious nut butter with either walnuts or almonds, instead of peanuts (see recipe on page 247).

Good to Know

Walnuts and almonds contain the highest levels of vitamin E of any food, except for certain vegetable oils.

Wheat

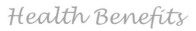

Anyone who is at all interested in the healing and health-giving properties of food should include wheat germ in their diet. Wheat germ is the embryo of a grain of wheat, and, as such, contains the essence of the whole plant—its vital center that is rich in vitamins and minerals. Wheat germ is also an important source of folic acid, zinc, magnesium, niacin, phosphorus, iron and copper, and it contains a very high amount of vitamin E.

Health Benefits

- Helps in fetal development
- Helps prevent cardiovascular disease
- Improves digestion
- Reduces the risk of cancer

Put To Good Use

People suffering from anemia are advised to eat 1 to 3 tsp (5 to 15 ml) of wheat germ daily, or to simply sprinkle it on their morning cereal or yogurt for two weeks every two or three months.

Caution

Wheat may cause certain allergies, notably celiac disease, which is an allergic reaction in the intestines to the gluten in wheat and several other grains.

Selecting & Storing

To ensure its freshness, try to smell the wheat germ before buying. It should have a pleasing odor of roasted grain. As with breadcrumbs, wheat germ can be frozen for up to six months in a sealed plastic bag. It does not need to be thawed before using.

Culinary Use

Sprinkle wheat germ on breakfast cereals, yogurt and meat stews, or use it when breading chicken or fish.

Recipes

- Homemade Granola (page 139)
- Homemade Muesli (page 143)

Healthful Hints

In meatloaf and meatball recipes, replace breadcrumbs with a mixture of oatmeal and wheat germ.

Beauty Secret

Lotion for extra-dry skin

In a double boiler, melt 1 oz (30 g) of beeswax in ⅓ cup (75 ml) of wheat germ oil. Add 4 drops of geranium rosat essential oil and 1 tsp (5 ml) of lemon juice. Stir well and pour into one or two small glass jars. The lotion stores well in a cool, dry place for up to three weeks. Apply to dry skin in the evening as a cold cream.

Good To Know

Adding a daily spoonful of wheat germ to your diet is tantamount to taking a vitamin E supplement. It is an efficient way of fortifying the body against cardiovascular disease and cancer.

Yogurt

As long as the yogurt you buy is free of additives and is unsweetened, it is an excellent food for your health. Yogurt is high in calcium, phosphorus and potassium, as well as vitamins A and B. The bacteria found in yogurt have the ability to prevent fungal infections (mycosis) and stimulate beneficial bacteria in the body to help destroy harmful ones.

Health Benefits

- Helps combat mild food poisoning
- Helps digestion
- Helps prevent infection
- Relieves stomach ulcers
- Stimulates the immune system

Put To Good Use

It is recommended that we eat one portion of plain yogurt daily, since it contains 40 percent of the recommended daily amount of calcium. Yogurt is also highly beneficial—and is often recommended by doctors—after a treatment involving antibiotics, to restore the natural flora (bacteria) in the digestive tract needed for proper digestion.

Caution

Keep in mind that, after a week or so, the active bacterial content of yogurt diminishes. To take advantage of all the health-giving properties of yogurt, it should be eaten within a few days of purchase.

Selecting & Storing

Avoid sweetened yogurts and those with added flavors, chemical colorings, preservatives and gelatin. Read the label carefully and, if you wish to eat fruit-flavored yogurt, choose a product with fruit at the top of the ingredients list. The best choice is organic yogurt.

Culinary Use

Yogurt is the ideal food partner at breakfast time, and it also makes for a delicious snack with added fresh fruits. It is irreplaceable in its ability to mellow spicy stews and curries, and it is a healthy alternative to sour cream or mayonnaise. It is also excellent in cold sauces and dips.

Recipes

- Budwig Cream (page 137)
- Curried Yogurt Dip with Pineapple (page 226)
- Fruit Trio Appetizer (page 137)
- Papaya Shrimp Salad with Kiwi (page 158)
- Tofu Mayonnaise (page 224)
- Yogurt Granola Cup with Nectarine (page 143)

Healthful Hints

Yogurt cheese

To make a delicious thickened yogurt, place plain yogurt in a strainer lined with cheesecloth and leave to drip overnight in the refrigerator.

Good To Know

Because yogurt does not tolerate heat and quickly loses its health-giving benefits, it should be added to hot dishes only at the very end of cooking.

Zucchini

The zucchini is the best-known summer squash in North America, though the flat, round pattypan squash and the more pear-shaped, yellow summer squash are two other varieties that deserve attention. All of these summer squash are eaten whole, and all have a mild flavor, are easy to digest and are a good source of fiber and vitamins A and C.

Health Benefits

- Aids digestion
- Helps protect against several types of cancer

Put To Good Use

Zucchini or Summer squash (unpeeled) alongside a meat dish will help digestion.

Caution

While zucchini is safe for most people, individuals with Oral Allergy Syndrome (see page 86) may have a reaction.

Selecting & Storing

Choose deep green zucchinis that seem heavy. Pattypan squash should be bright yellow without blemishes. Yellow squash should be firm with a smooth skin. They all keep well in the refrigerator.

Culinary Use

Zucchini is used in all sorts of delicious recipes: soups, appetizers, baked vegetables dishes *au gratin*, salads, cakes and muffins. Yellow squash is almost as versatile, though not used for desserts. Pattypan squash is usually cooked as a stuffed squash in the oven.

Recipes

- Parsnip and Zucchini Soup (page 169)
- Ratatouille Niçoise (page 155)
- Spaghetti with Meatless... Sauce (page 206)
- Zucchini Buckwheat Loaf Cake (page 238)
- Zucchini Chocolate Loaf Cake (page 237)
- Zucchini Soup (page 170)

Healthful Hints

The flesh of the zucchini adds body to a soup and is a healthier alternative to the potato as a thickener.

Good To Know

Gray and white zucchinis are a variety with green flesh inside and a whitish skin. They tend to be larger than regular zucchini, and, like their smaller green cousin, can be stuffed and baked in the oven.

Part Two

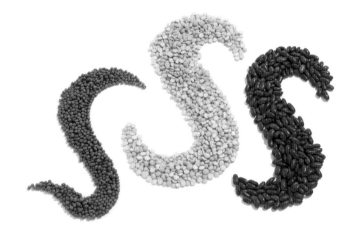

The Motto for Healthy Eating
Healthy · Simple · Delicious

Cooking is way of intimately participating in the maintenance of our health and well being. When we take the time to cook, our sensory relationship established with the food—by sight, texture, manipulation, aroma and taste—brings us into closer contact with our deeper, basic needs. This heightened connection with food during the cooking process brings many people to a new understanding and recognition of the specific foods they have discovered that make them feel healthy and well. There is nothing particularly mysterious about this attitude towards the food we prepare and eat; indeed it springs naturally from a better awareness of the close connection between our food and our health.

Even if you have not yet discovered the pleasure of including these healing foods into your diet (and appreciating their benefits), you will have no difficulty preparing the straightforward recipes presented here. Each dish has been conceived to respect the three words of our motto for better eating: healthy, simple and delicious. All of the recipes have been created so as to make best use of the 86 healing foods listed in Part One. Each recipe also keeps two things in mind: to bring out all of the therapeutic value of the foods, and to bring out the unique flavors of each ingredient. Grouped in a way that best allows you to create entire menus for each day of the week, these recipes will help you put into practice what you have learned in Part One about the extraordinary—and completely natural—medicinal properties of various foods, and the importance of eating a wide variety of them each day to create a well-balanced diet.

Food Choices

If your health has become a major concern in your life, and you have become preoccupied with preserving or improving it at all costs, you are probably among the growing number of people buying **organic foods**—foods that are not treated with chemical pesticides or preservatives. Even if you have not yet considered switching to organic, you should still work towards increasing your intake of fresh fruits, vegetables and grains without fear of contamination. Governments and health experts are confident that the wholesome healing foods listed in this book generally contain only negligible quantities of residues, with very minimal risk of affecting our health. Washing fruits and vegetables well under running water before eating will generally reduce all risks associated with bacteria or chemicals.

To take best advantage of the benefits of a given food, it is important to choose **fresh produce** wherever possible, in its most natural state. While frozen vegetables might seem practical, most, unfortunately, do not retain their health-giving properties. The processing required to freeze or can fruits and vegetables involves exposure to heat and water, which often has the effect of removing many precious nutrients. When heated or boiled, for example, a fair amount of the insoluble fiber of many vegetables is converted to soluble fiber, and the levels of potassium are basically lost. As for vitamin content, processing often causes a loss of between 10 and 40 percent. If it is impossible for you to obtain fresh fruits and vegetables during some seasons of the year, get into the habit of freezing your own produce in season. This is done quite simply after blanching them in boiling water for a minute or two.

To enhance the flavors of a meal and to better develop the taste of individual foods, nothing works better than adding **fine herbs**. Most herbs have medicinal properties as well—all the more reason to include them. The majority of supermarkets now offer fresh herbs such as basil, mint, tarragon, coriander, sage and thyme; many all year round. In summer, however, it is fairly easy and rewarding to plant your own herb garden, even on a windowsill or balcony. Spices also play an essential role in cooking. Try to buy spices in bulk-food shops, measuring out only the quantities you need (preferably whole, un-ground), then grind and prepare your own mixtures, taking care to label your containers. Your meals will become more varied and in the end you will actually save time and money. To prepare your own herb and spice mixtures, take a look at the recipes offered in the section Beverages and Other Preparations on page 243.

Meal Preparation

In this book we have chosen not to give meal suggestions since we feel that you are the person best suited to make such decisions. Only you know which dishes are best for you at any given time, according to your tastes and health needs. You know best your own state of health and, after having read in Part One about the healing properties of a variety of foods, only you will know which types of foods and dishes will best help you to restore your health or protect against disease. You are in the best position to make these choices. That said, you should not suddenly start to eat a lot of one type of food that you are unaccustomed to—especially if you are eating it to treat a health condition—without first consulting a medical professional or nutrition specialist. What we need to understand is that it is a wide variety of healing foods in our diet that will give us the greatest benefits towards maintaining good health. If you discover an unfamiliar food that you would like to try including in your diet, do so gradually and never consume any food excessively, particularly in the first few days. As we emphasized on several occasions in Part One, it is important to take care when adding new foods to our diet, and those foods should be eaten in moderation. Prudence and moderation are always the best rules when it comes to matters of nutrition.

Basic Equipment

A huge arsenal of sophisticated, expensive cookware is really not required in order to cook well. All you need are two or three saucepans, a baking sheet, a roasting pan, a large pot, an electric blender, an electric grinder and a few sharp kitchen knives. An electric food processor is not mandatory, but is handy for two or three of the recipes included here. What are most important, apart from your ten fingers, are your taste buds…and your desire to explore the new foods, new tastes and new textures, all of which will help bring you improved health and well being.

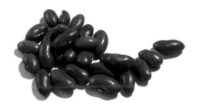

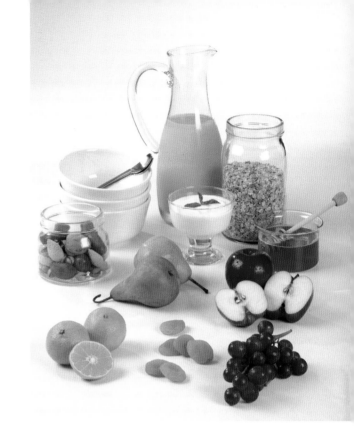

Breakfast

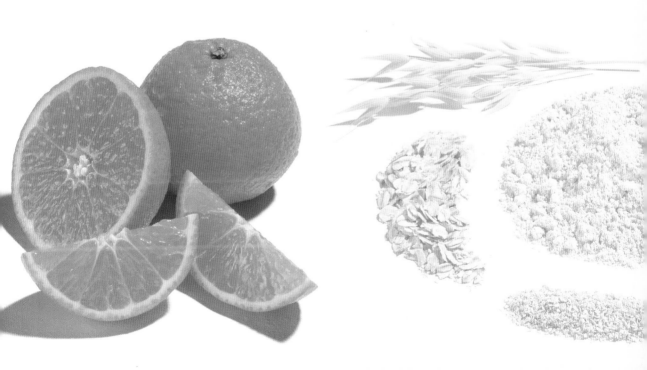

Hearty Breakfasts

According to a proverb made popular by a certain weight-loss expert, to lose weight without compromising your health, one should "eat like a king at breakfast, like a prince at lunchtime, and like a beggar for supper." Though this idea makes good sense, it still seems contrary to many of our customs and habits, and if you really want to put it into practice, it might require major changes to your morning routine. No dietician or specialist in nutrition will dispute the evidence supporting the fact that breakfast should be the most substantial meal of the day. Though not necessarily the largest meal, it should be the most nutritious and vitamin-rich, prepared in such a way that it supplies all of the nutrients the body needs to function properly.

The best way to begin the day is to enjoy a dish of Budwig Cream (page 137), a unique formula that possesses, among other merits, all of the most important nutrients for the body. Easy to prepare, this breakfast food is truly delectable.

For people who cannot even manage the extra five to ten minutes needed to make this tasty breakfast food, any well-balanced breakfast should contain fruits, cereals and dairy products. Fruit can be in the form of juice or fresh fruits eaten raw. Juice has the advantage of perhaps combining the benefits of several different fruits—a bonus for those seeking a very well-balanced offering of vitamins. If you have only a few minutes each day to prepare a complete breakfast, a juicer may be a worthwhile investment. You can also make do with simply eating two or three different fruits, a handful of almonds and a small bowl of yogurt: a basic formula that will very adequately prepare you for your day's activities.

Pre-packaged breakfast cereals found in every supermarket are generally over-sweetened and full of food additives. It is actually very easy—and more economical—to prepare your own granola or cereal mixtures, and to complement these with dried fruits and nuts. The homemade cereals proposed in this section will store well for weeks in the refrigerator, and you can enjoy them any time: as a dessert or snack, served with milk or soy drink, with yogurt or cottage cheese.

Breakfast Recipes

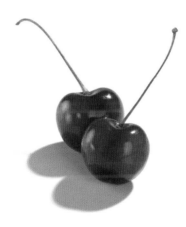

Orange and Cherry Soy Smoothie

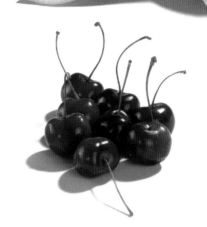

The vitamin C from the orange, the antioxidants of the cherries and the cancer-fighting compounds of the soybean make this beverage a powerful health drink to start your day off right.

Ingredients *(4 servings)*

2 oranges, peeled and cut into pieces
zest of 1 orange
20 fresh cherries, pitted
1 cup (250 ml) soy milk
honey, to taste

Instructions

- Put all ingredients in a blender and mix well.
- Serve in fruit or ice-cream cups and garnish with more cherries.

Apricot, Fig and Clementine Purée

Served with frozen yogurt, this purée is naturally sweetened and makes for a refreshing dessert. High in dietary fiber, it is a fortifying and rejuvenating mixture with preventive properties, that goes very well with whole grain toast at breakfast time.

Ingredients *(4 servings)*

½ cup (125 ml) dried figs, chopped, with stems removed
½ cup (125 ml) dried apricots, chopped
1 ¼ cup (310 ml) water
6 whole kernels Jamaican allspice
1 tsp (5 ml) ginger, freshly grated
grated zest and juice of ½ lemon
2 clementines, peeled and cut into pieces

Instructions

- Put figs and apricots in a saucepan with water, allspice, ginger and lemon juice, and bring to a boil.
- Cover, reduce heat and let simmer for 20 minutes until the fruits have softened.
- Add lemon zest and allow to cool.
- Add clementines and mix well. Refrigerate.
- Serve the purée cold or at room temperature. Keeps for about five days in the refrigerator.

Fresh Grape Jam

This delicious, flavorful jam will keep for several weeks in the refrigerator.

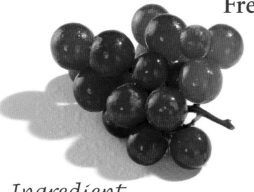

Instructions

- Combine all ingredients in a stainless steel or enamel saucepan, and bring to a boil.
- Reduce heat and let simmer for 1 ½ hours, or until grapes become a rich color and a spoonful of the liquid thickens on a plate. (This thickened syrup forms in the final half-hour, so be careful to watch for this final stage of cooking.)
- Allow to cool, then pour into glass jars, leaving a 1-inch (2.5-cm) space from the top.
- Seal each jar with a lid. The jam keeps for about one month in the refrigerator, or six months in the freezer.

Ingredient

2 ½ lb (1 kg) red grapes, washed, pitted, sliced in half
3 cups (750 ml) sugar
½ cup (125 ml) apple cider vinegar
¼ cup (60 ml) water
2 slices of lemon, seeds removed
1 tsp (5 ml) whole cloves

Apple, Pear and Prune Purée

Naturally sweetened, this fruit purée is delicious at breakfast time, served with whole grain toast or crackers.

Ingredients

½ cup (125 ml) prunes, pitted
1 cup (250 ml) pineapple juice
3 ripe pears, peeled and cut into pieces
3 apples, peeled and cut into pieces
zest of 1 orange

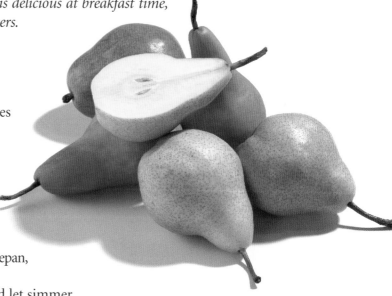

Instructions

- Soak prunes in pineapple juice for four hours.
- Heat prunes and juice gently in a saucepan, then add remaining ingredients.
- Bring to a boil, then lower heat and let simmer for 30 minutes. Serve warm or cold.

Fruit Trio Appetizer

This combination of delicious fruits makes for a nutritious breakfast or an energizing snack.

Ingredients *(2 servings)*

1 grapefruit, peeled with seeds removed, cut into bite-size pieces
1 ripe banana, sliced
24 cherries, pitted
juice of 1 orange (freshly squeezed) with the orange's grated zest
½ cup (125 ml) plain yogurt
flaked almonds to garnish

Instructions

- Mix the fruits in a bowl. Divide to fill two fruit cups.
- Sprinkle with orange juice and zest.
- Top with yogurt and garnish with almond slivers. Serve immediately.

Budwig Cream

Created and popularized by the prominent Swiss doctor, Catherine Kousmine, who gained her reputation by focusing on food to treat serious illnesses, this recipe packs a whole array of ingredients necessary for good health into a single breakfast dish.

Ingredients *(2 servings)*

¼ cup (60 ml) buckwheat grains
¼ cup (60 ml) flaxseed
18 almonds
½ cup (125 ml) plain yogurt
¼ cup (60 ml) sunflower oil
juice of ½ lemon
2 tbsp (30 ml) honey
1 chopped apple or sliced banana

Instructions

- Finely grind buckwheat grains in a coffee grinder. Set aside.
- Repeat with the flaxseed. Then grind the almonds more coarsely. Combine these three ingredients in a bowl and set aside.
- In a second bowl, beat together the yogurt and oil. Add lemon juice and honey, then the fruit and the grain mixture.
- Serve immediately.

Buckwheat Pancakes

These little pancakes are quick and easy to prepare. Highly digestible, they can also be enjoyed by those with an intolerance to gluten.

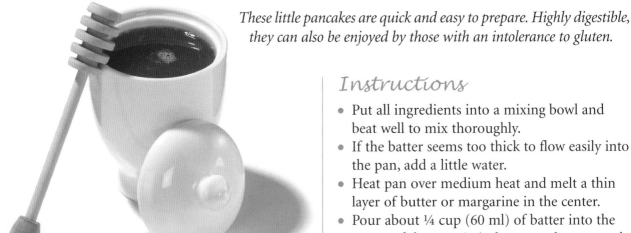

Instructions

- Put all ingredients into a mixing bowl and beat well to mix thoroughly.
- If the batter seems too thick to flow easily into the pan, add a little water.
- Heat pan over medium heat and melt a thin layer of butter or margarine in the center.
- Pour about ¼ cup (60 ml) of batter into the center of the pan. Swivel pan gently to spread out the batter. As soon as bubbles begin to reach the surface of the pancake and edges are cooked, turn it over and cook for another 30 to 60 seconds.
- These pancakes are delicious served with yogurt, jam, fruit purée or honey.

Ingredients *(8 pancakes)*

1 cup (250 ml) buckwheat flour
1 ¼ cups (310 ml) water
½ tsp (2 ml) salt
¼ tsp (1 ml) baking soda
¼ tsp (1 ml) baking powder
butter or non-hydrogenated margarine for frying

Sweet Variation

- Add 2 tbsp (30 ml) of brown sugar or honey, the grated zest of 1 orange and a pinch of nutmeg to the batter before cooking.

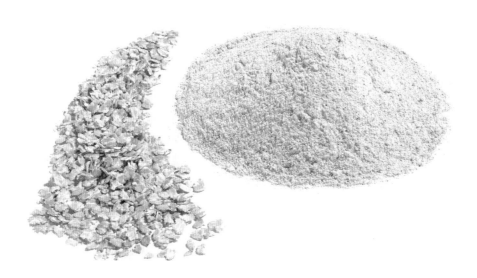

Soy Milk with Mango

This drink can be made quickly and is a healthy, vitamin-rich substitute for your morning glass of orange juice. As well as being rich in vitamins A and C, it helps to rejuvenate the cells. Its rich texture makes for a snack drink that children will love.

Ingredients *(2 servings)*

1 ripe mango, peeled, pitted and cut into bite-size pieces
1 cup (250 ml) plain or vanilla-flavored soy milk
fresh mint leaves for garnish

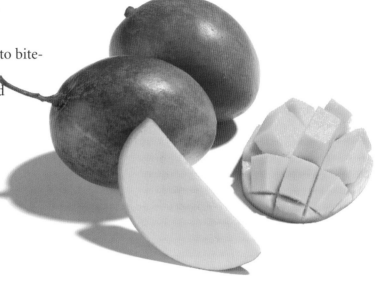

Instructions

- Blend mango and soy milk to a creamy consistency in a blender.
- Serve in pretty fruit cups and garnish with mint.

Homemade Granola

The possibilities are endless as to the mixture of grains, nuts and dried fruits you can use to make granola. Feel free to experiment with your own healthy combinations. Below is a basic mixture that is nutritious, delicious and easy to prepare.

Ingredients

2 cups (500 ml) rolled oats or coarse oatmeal
½ cup (125 ml) rye or spelt flakes
½ cup (125 ml) wheat flakes
½ cup (125 ml) flaked almonds
½ cup (125 ml) shredded coconut
½ cup (125 ml) unsalted sunflower seeds
¼ cup (60 ml) wheat germ
½ tsp (2 ml) cinnamon
¼ cup (60 ml) honey
¼ cup (60 ml) grapeseed oil (or sunflower oil)

Instructions

- Preheat oven to 350ºF (180ºC).
- Mix together all dry ingredients in a large bowl.
- Gently heat together the honey and oil (30 seconds in the microwave is sufficient).
- Add the honey mixture to dry ingredients and mix well. Spread out on a cookie sheet.
- Bake for about 20 minutes, mixing halfway through cooking time. Cook until granola is golden brown.
- Leave to cool, then put in sealed containers. Will keep for up to three months in the refrigerator.

Buckwheat Muffins
with Apple and Beet

The tasty combination of flavors in these muffins is quite unique and not at all like the flavors of the uncooked base ingredients. Yet no flavor is lost or masked and none of the health-giving properties are diminished.

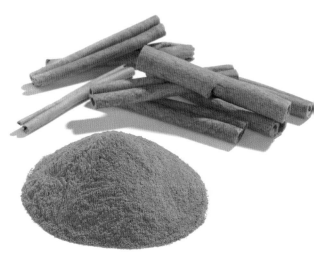

Ingredients *(8 muffins)*

½ cup (125 ml) buckwheat flour
¼ cup (60 ml) whole wheat flour
½ cup (125 ml) sugar
½ tsp (2 ml) baking soda
½ tsp (2 ml) baking powder
¼ tsp (1 ml) nutmeg
¼ tsp (1 ml) cinnamon
grated zest of ½ orange
½ cup (125 ml) grated beet (1 small beet)
¼ cup (60 ml) grated apple, peeled (1 small apple)
1 egg
⅓ cup (75 ml) grapeseed or sunflower oil
¼ cup (60 ml) unsalted sunflower seeds (optional)

Instructions

- Preheat oven to 350ºF (180ºC).
- Sift together the dry ingredients.
- Add the rest of the ingredients, mixing with a wooden spoon just enough to moisten (not more than 2 minutes).
- Pour batter into greased muffin tins.
- Bake for about 20 minutes.

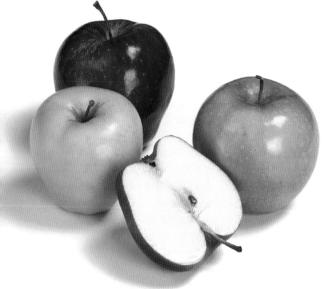

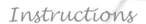

Bran Fig Muffins

These muffins have a lovely flavor of fig and molasses. Rich in calcium, they are a delicious protection against osteoporosis.

Ingredients *(1 dozen muffins)*

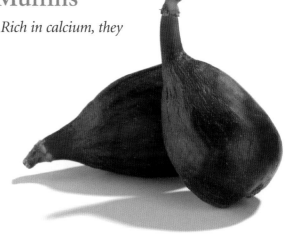

1 cup (250 ml) oat bran
½ cup (125 ml) all-purpose flour
½ cup (125 ml) wholewheat flour
3 tbsp (45 ml) sugar
¾ tsp (4 ml) baking soda
½ tsp (2 ml) salt
½ tsp (2 ml) cinnamon
1 large egg
¾ cup (180 ml) unsweetened evaporated milk
⅓ cup (75 ml) molasses
⅓ cup (75 ml) grapeseed or sunflower oil
¼ cup (60 ml) chopped dried figs (stems removed)
¼ cup (60 ml) raisins
grated zest of 1 orange

Instructions

- Preheat oven to 375ºF (190ºC).
- Mix oat bran, flours, sugar, baking soda, salt and cinnamon in a large bowl.
- Beat the egg in a second bowl. Beat in milk, molasses and oil.
- Mix in the dried fruits and orange zest.
- Pour the egg-fruit mixture into the dry mixture and stir just enough to moisten. Take care not to over-mix.
- Spoon batter into oiled or buttered muffin tins.
- Bake for 25 minutes or until a toothpick inserted into a muffin comes out clean.

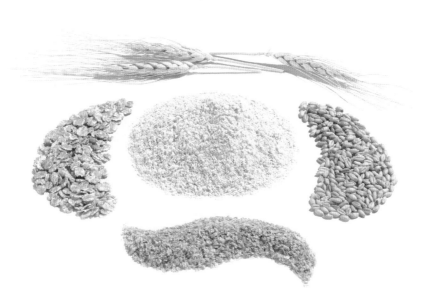

Almond Muffins

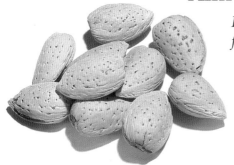

Light and delicious, these muffins have a nutty almond flavor and are a substantial, tasty breakfast treat.

Instructions

- Preheat oven to 375°F (190°C).
- Grease muffin tins with oil or butter.
- Put poppy seeds into a bowl, then sift in flour, baking powder and salt. Add sugar. Mix well and create a well in the center.
- Beat together the eggs and milk in a second bowl. Add the oil a little at a time, then the almond extract, ground almonds and orange zest. Mix together.
- Pour the liquid mixture into the center of the dry mixture. Do not over-mix; the batter should remain somewhat crumbly.
- Fill each muffin cup to ¾ full.
- Bake for 20 to 25 minutes or until a toothpick inserted into a muffin comes out clean.
- Allow to cool fully before removing from muffin tins.

Ingredients *(1 dozen muffins)*

2 tbsp (30 ml) poppy seeds (optional)
1 ¼ cups (310 ml) flour (half-half mixture of all-purpose and whole wheat)
2 tbsp (30 ml) baking powder
¼ tsp (1 ml) salt
½ cup (125 ml) sugar
2 eggs
1 cup (250 ml) milk
½ cup (125 ml) grapeseed or sunflower oil
½ tsp (2 ml) almond extract
¼ cup (60 ml) roasted almonds, ground
grated zest of 1 orange

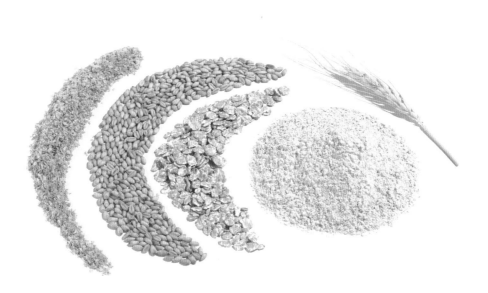

Homemade Muesli

This traditional Scandinavian mixture of grains is an excellent breakfast cereal that, thanks to its very high dietary fiber content, is an excellent protection against cardiovascular disease.

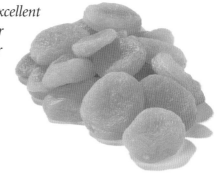

Ingredients *(4 - 6 servings)*

3 cups (750 ml) rolled oat flakes (not 'instant' oats)
½ cup (125 ml) dried apricots, chopped
½ cup (125 ml) dates or dried apples, chopped
½ cup (125 ml) oat bran
½ cup (125 ml) unsalted sunflower seeds
½ cup (125 ml) raisins
¼ cup (60 ml) wheat bran
¼ cup (60 ml) wheat germ

Instructions

- In a large bowl, mix together all the muesli ingredients. Pour into a sealed plastic container and refrigerate. Will keep for several weeks in the refrigerator.

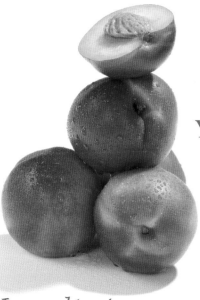

Yogurt Granola Cup with Nectarine

Most fruit-flavored yogurt sold in the supermarket is overly sweetened with sugar. Try this combination that is garnished with honey and crunchy granola. Children will love it for breakfast or as a snack.

Ingredients *(4 servings)*

¾ cup (180 ml) plain yogurt
2 tbsp (30 ml) honey
¼ cup (60 ml) Homemade Granola (see page 139)
4 nectarines, fully ripe, peeled and cut into bite-size pieces
20 strawberries, sliced

Instructions

- Mix yogurt and honey in a small bowl. Set aside.
- In a blender, purée nectarines, then add half the yogurt mixture. Mix again.
- Pour yogurt-nectarine mixture into four serving cups.
- Cover each cup with 1 tbsp (15 ml) of granola.
- Divide the remaining yogurt-honey mixture equally into each cup and garnish with slices of strawberry.

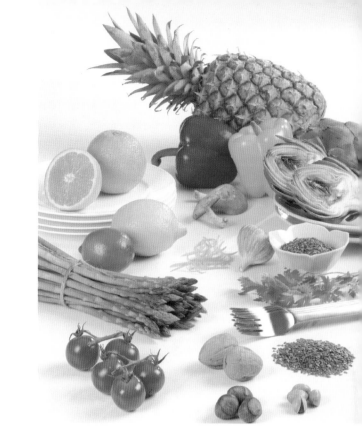

Appetizers

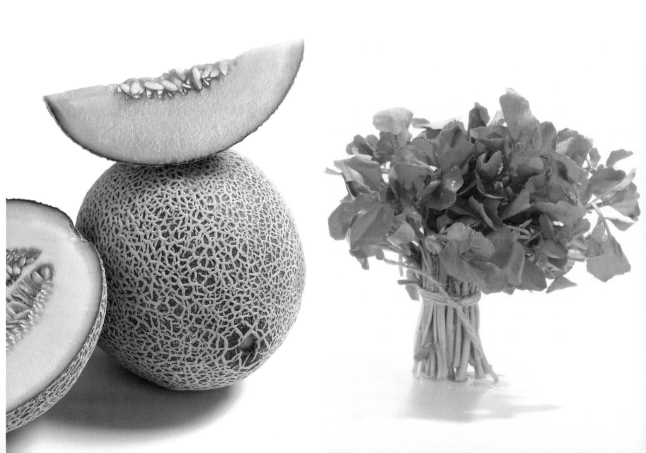

Appetizing Appetizers

The rule of thumb that we have chosen to follow in our choice of appetizers is flavor over fullness. Appetizers should stimulate the appetite and prepare us for the meal to follow without trying to fill or weigh down the stomach. Appetizers should tantalize the palate, inviting our dinner guests to make way for a lovely meal. With this in mind, the best combinations of foods are tasteful contrasts, such as the acidity of certain fruits paired with energy-rich vegetables—mixtures of flavors that are simultaneously astonishing and delicious. Fresh herbs and the zest of oranges and lemons all play key roles in enhancing and developing the flavors and aromas of these dishes. It is for this reason that we have included several refreshing salads with unexpected flavorings among the appetizer choices that follow.

Appetizer Recipes

(continued)

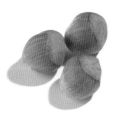

Pineapple Guacamole

This attractive and flavorful combination of vitamin-rich fruits will help the elimination of "bad" (LDL) cholesterol when served before a meal of red meat.

Ingredients *(4 servings)*

1 tbsp (15 ml) lime juice
3 tbsp (45 ml) olive oil
a dash of Harissa Chili Sauce (see page 223) or Tabasco sauce
1 small bunch of coriander (cilantro) leaves, chopped
8 slices of fresh pineapple, cut into triangles
1 mango, peeled and cut into bite-size pieces
1 ripe avocado, cut into bite-size pieces and sprinkled with lime juice
salt and pepper to taste

Instructions

- Combine salt and lime juice in a salad bowl. Add oil and Harissa sauce and mix together well. Adjust seasoning.
- Add coriander leaves and mix again.
- Blend in the fruits, mixing carefully. Serve immediately.

Artichokes with Garlic and Lemon
(microwave recipe)

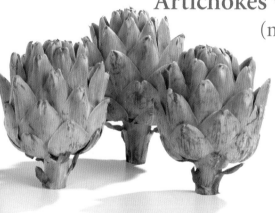

This is a simple and delicious way to get the best from artichokes, which are excellent for the liver. Even better, the garlic and lemon juice possess potent antiviral properties.

Instructions

- Prepare artichokes by cutting off the stems and removing the small leaves at the base. Rinse in cold water.
- Place each artichoke in a baking dish or ramekin just large enough to contain the vegetable. Add 2 tbsp (30 ml) water to each.
- Cover each baking dish with plastic wrap but do not seal it completely.
- Cook for 12 to 15 minutes.*
- While the artichokes cool, prepare the vinaigrette by mixing the garlic, lemon juice and olive oil. Drizzle artichokes with vinaigrette and serve.

Ingredients *(4 servings)*

4 artichokes
¼ cup (60 ml) olive oil
2 tbsp (30 ml) lemon juice
2 garlic cloves, minced

* Cooking time for 1 artichoke: 5-7 min.; 2 artichokes: 10-11 min.; 3 or 4 artichokes: 12-15 min.

Asparagus in Curry Sauce à l'Orange

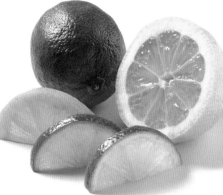

This delicate, warm appetizer is particularly recommended for people suffering from kidney afflictions.

Ingredients *(4 servings)*

2 tbsp (30 ml) butter
1 small shallot, minced
1 small clove of garlic, minced
1 tbsp (15 ml) flour
1 tsp (5 ml) curry powder
⅓ cup (75 ml) orange juice
zest of 1 orange
⅓ cup (75 ml) chicken broth (see page 165)
⅓ cup (75 ml) table cream (15%)
1 tbsp (15 ml) coriander leaves, finely chopped
1 bunch asparagus

Instruction

- Melt the butter in a small saucepan, and brown the shallot for 1 or 2 minutes. Add garlic and cook 1 minute more.
- Add flour and mix well.
- Add curry powder, orange juice, zest and broth. Cook for a few minutes until sauce begins to thicken.
- Add cream, then coriander. Remove from heat and allow to cool.
- Meanwhile, cook asparagus in boiling water for 4 minutes; they should remain firm and crunchy.
- Drain and arrange on a serving dish. Drizzle curry sauce over the asparagus.

Sardine Canapés

A refreshing appetizer, rich in protein and vitamins.

Ingredients *(2 to 4 servings)*

1 can of sardines, drained
1 tbsp (15 ml) Egg-Free Mayonnaise (see recipe on page 224)
1 small clove of garlic, minced
1 small shallot, minced
zest of ½ lemon
2 tbsp (30 ml) dill sprigs, chives or parsley

Instructions

- In a small bowl, crush the sardines with a fork. Mix in the mayonnaise, garlic and shallot.
- Add lemon zest and herbs, and mix again.
- Serve on crackers or rye crisp breads.

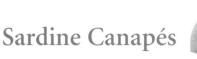

Cantaloupe with Chèvre and Porto

This elegant, vitamin-rich appetizer offers a delicate marriage of flavors while bringing together a fine combination of health-giving foods.

Ingredients *(4 servings)*

1 small cantaloupe
¼ cup (60 ml) Porto
⅓ lb (150 g) fine chèvre (goat's milk) cheese
lettuce leaves and fresh basil or mint, for garnish

Instructions

- Halve the melon, remove and discard seeds.
- Using a small, round spoon, cut out bite-size pieces of melon and arrange in a mixing bowl.
- Pour over the Porto and allow to marinate for 15 minutes.

- Cut the cheese into cubes, add to melon and carefully mix together well.
- Line the bottom of four dessert bowls or ramekins with the lettuce leaves.
- Add the cantaloupe and cheese mixture to the bowls and garnish with basil or mint leaves.

Carrots and Parsnips with Dulse

This delectable appetizer is a refreshing new way to include seaweed in your diet, so as to benefit from its anti-rheumatic and anti-bacterial therapeutic properties.

Instructions

- Rehydrate dried dulse by soaking in warm water for 3 minutes. Drain, air-dry and chop.
- Blend all ingredients in a bowl. Chill for 1 hour in the refrigerator before serving.

Variations

- Replace the parsnip or carrot with grated celeriac (celery root) or finely chopped cabbage; replace the lemon juice with apple cider vinegar; replace the parsley with coriander, and add to this salad canned lentils or chick peas to make an appetizer full of revitalizing and anti-viral properties.

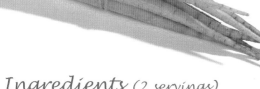

Ingredients *(2 servings)*

1 medium carrot, grated
1 small parsnip, grated
1 tbsp (15 ml) dried dulse
2 tbsp (30 ml) fresh parsley, chopped
1 tbsp (15 ml) lemon juice
2 tbsp (30 ml) olive oil
1 tbsp (15 ml) sesame seeds

Stuffed Mushrooms

Garlic and parsley come together in this delicious appetizer—two ingredients highly recommended for people suffering from anemia.

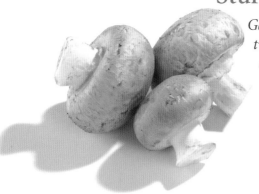

Ingredients *(4 servings)*

12 medium mushrooms with stems
2 cloves of garlic, minced
2 tbsp (30 ml) clarified butter* or non-hydrogenated margarine
2 tbsp (30 ml) parsley, chopped
12 pistachios, shelled and chopped
fresh young spinach or lettuce

Instructions

- Preheat oven to 425ºF (220ºC).
- Remove stems from mushrooms and wash.
- Chop stems finely and mix with garlic, clarified butter, parsley and pistachios.
- Stuff each mushroom with this mixture and arrange in ramekin dishes.
- Bake until butter begins to bubble on the surface of the mushrooms.
- Remove from oven, allow to cool slightly and arrange on a bed of salad leaves. Serve with slices of crunchy French bread.

* To make a quick and easy clarified butter, melt butter in a small pan, allow to cool slightly and skim off the milky deposits floating at the surface.

Spinach and Tomato *au Gratin*

This mouth-watering dish is prepared in a flash and is full of healing nutrients with properties that protect against viral infections.

Ingredients *(4 servings)*

1 package of fresh spinach, carefully washed, stems removed
1 tbsp (15 ml) clarified butter (see above)
¼ tsp (1 ml) ground nutmeg
2 cloves of garlic, minced
2 fresh tomatoes, seeded and crushed
3 tbsp (45 ml) mixture of breadcrumbs and ground pecans
salt and pepper
1 egg, beaten
¼ cup (60 ml) grated Parmesan cheese

Instruction

- Preheat oven to 375ºF (190ºC).
- Melt butter in large saucepan, add spinach and nutmeg, cover.
- Lower heat immediately and stir spinach to coat leaves in butter and nutmeg. As soon as spinach leaves are soft, drain excess butter and arrange on a baking dish. Season with salt and pepper.
- Add garlic and tomatoes, season again and mix all ingredients together.
- Sprinkle with the breadcrumb-pecan mixture.
- Beat together the egg and Parmesan cheese. Pour over spinach-tomato dish.
- Bake for about 10 minutes.

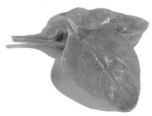

Fillet of Raw Salmon with Herb Salt

This delicate and refined appetizer is an easy dinner party dish that can be prepared the night before. It contains a healthy amount of omega-3 fatty acids, compounds that are vital for the efficient functioning of the cardiovascular system, the brain and the glands.

Ingredients *(4 servings)*

¾-lb (350-g) fillet of very fresh salmon
zest and juice of 1 lemon
1 tbsp (15 ml) mixed herbs to which ½ tsp (2 ml) of salt has been added
1 tsp (5 ml) ground fennel seeds
2 tbsp (30 ml) fresh dill, chopped
1 tsp (5 ml) olive oil

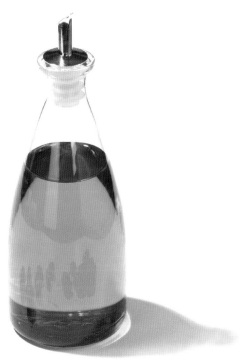

Instructions

- Carefully wash the salmon fillet. Pat dry.
- Mix together the zest and juice of the lemon, the herb salt, fennel, dill and olive oil. Set aside.
- Using a very sharp knife, cut salmon into thin slices.
- In a large shallow dish, arrange salmon slices to cover the bottom, then drizzle with herb-lemon juice mixture. Add another layer of salmon and drizzle again. Repeat as necessary.
- Cover dish with plastic wrap and refrigerate for about 6 hours.
- Twist salmon slices into rosette shapes and serve cold on rye crackers or crisp breads.

Variation

- The salmon fillet can be chopped instead of sliced, then mixed carefully with the herb – lemon juice mixture. The chopped, marinated salmon should be divided and put into single-serving ramekins, covered in plastic wrap and refrigerated for 6 hours or more. These ramekins can then be simply turned over and served on a bed of cress or spinach leaves.

Mushroom and Walnut Spread

This delicious spread is flavored with lemon and coriander and makes for a lovely appetizer that also helps to lower levels of "bad" (LDL) cholesterol.

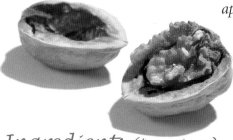

Ingredients *(4 servings)*

¼ cup (60 ml) non-hydrogenated margarine
1 shallot, chopped
8-oz (227-g) package of white, brown or mixed mushrooms, chopped
1 tbsp (15 ml) tahini*
1 small clove of garlic, minced
1 tsp (5 ml) lemon juice
zest of ½ lemon
2-3 drops Harissa Chili Sauce (see page 223)
¼ cup (60 ml) walnuts, pecans or pistachios, chopped
1 bunch coriander leaves, chopped
salt and pepper

Instructions

- In a saucepan, sauté the shallot in 1 tbsp (15 ml) of the margarine, without browning.
- Add mushrooms and garlic. Cook for 10 minutes until cooking liquid has evaporated.
- Remove from heat and allow to cool.
- Add the lemon juice and zest, Harissa sauce, remaining margarine, tahini, chopped nuts and coriander leaves.
- Season with salt and pepper. Put mixture in blender and mix briefly so that some chunks remain.
- Pour into a baking dish or ramekins, cover with plastic wrap and refrigerate for at least 12 hours.
- Serve on rye bread, crackers or crisp breads.

* Tahini is a purée made from sesame seeds, found in many specialty and health food shops.

Flaxseed Spread

Quick to prepare (aside from the soaking time of the seeds), this appetizer is rich in omega-3 fatty acids. Served on rice crackers or rye crisp bread, and accompanied by raw vegetables, this appetizer is a refreshing, healthier alternative to cold cuts or pâté de foie gras.

Ingredients

½ cup (125 ml) pumpkin seeds
½ cup (125 ml) unsalted sunflower seeds
¼ cup (60 ml) flaxseed, whole or ground
1 tbsp (15 ml) olive oil
½ tsp (2 ml) fennel seeds, crushed
1 tsp (5 ml) fresh ginger, grated
¼ tsp (1 ml) mustard powder
¼ cup (60 ml) cream cheese
salt and pepper

Instructions

- Soak pumpkin and sunflower seeds for at least 3 hours.
- If whole, grind the flaxseed and set aside.
- Put all of the ingredients into a blender. Mix to a smooth consistency.
- Taste, adjust seasoning and add more oil if necessary.

Lentil Terrines with Mushroom

These tasty terrines have complex flavors and seasonings that make them an excellent cold appetizer served on rye crisps or sesame crackers.

Ingredients *(4 terrines)*

2 tbsp (30 ml) butter or non-hydrogenated margarine
1 shallot, minced
8-oz (227-g) package of mushrooms, chopped
1 small clove of garlic, minced
2 tbsp (30 ml) Porto
1 ⅓ cups (325 ml) cooked lentils, rinsed and drained
1 egg, beaten
¼ cup (60 ml) bread crumbs (or mixture of crushed crackers and ground nuts)
1 tsp (5 ml) dried basil
½ tsp (2 ml) ground fennel seeds
½ tsp (2 ml) ground coriander seeds
2 tbsp (30 ml) fresh parsley, chopped
salt and pepper

Instructions

- Preheat oven to 350ºF (180ºC).
- In a saucepan, melt the butter and brown the shallot, mushrooms and garlic for 10 minutes.
- Let cool, then transfer to a blender and add cooked lentils. Process for 1 or 2 minutes to make a rich mixture that still has some texture. Set aside.
- Mix together the beaten egg, breadcrumbs and mushroom-lentil mixture in a bowl. Add the herbs, spices and parsley. Mix well and transfer to 4 ramekins (or terrine dishes).
- Bake for 35 minutes.

Ratatouille Niçoise

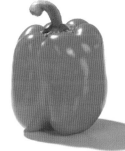

This appetizer is especially delicious in the fall. It is full of colorful vegetables with cancer-fighting properties.

Ingredients *(4 servings)*

3 tbsp (45 ml) olive oil
2 red or orange sweet peppers
2 onions, chopped
4 large ripe tomatoes, seeded and crushed (or 2 cups / 500 ml) of canned crushed tomatoes)
1 eggplant, sliced and cubed
2 zucchinis, sliced and cubed
4 cloves of garlic, minced
1 tsp (5 ml) mixed herbs Provençal (marjoram, thyme, basil, rosemary, savory)
¼ cup (60 ml) fresh basil leaves, chopped
salt and pepper

Instructions

- Brown the onions and peppers in the oil in a large pot over medium heat.
- Add the tomatoes, eggplant, zucchini, garlic, herbs, salt and pepper.
- Bring to a boil, then reduce heat and simmer for 30 minutes.
- Add the basil, remove from heat and let sit for 15 minutes before serving. This ratatouille is best when given time to allow the flavors to develop. It therefore improves upon reheating, and can be frozen for several months.

Beet and Carrot Salad

The mixture of ginger and cinnamon flavors combined with the delicate raw beet will impress your dinner guests. Served as an appetizer, it tantalizes the taste buds while helping with digestion and preventing anemia.

Ingredients *(4 servings)*

2 medium beets, peeled and grated
3 large carrots, scrubbed and grated
½ cup (125 ml) unsalted sunflower seeds
1 tsp (5 ml) fresh ginger, grated
½ tsp (2 ml) cinnamon
3 tbsp (45 ml) olive oil
1 tbsp (15 ml) apple cider vinegar
salt and pepper

Instructions

- Mix together the grated vegetables and sunflower seeds in a large bowl, then stir in the remaining ingredients.
- Serve. This salad will taste just as good the next day, having been refrigerated overnight.

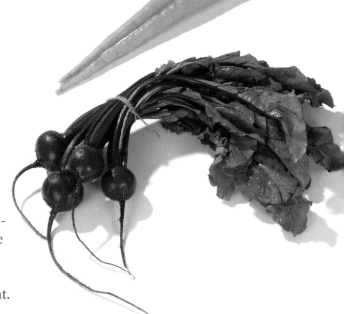

Cress Salad with Apple, Hazelnut and Chèvre

An invigorating and fortifying salad made with ingredients that help prevent cancer.

Ingredients *(4 servings)*

1 bunch of cress
2 fresh Empire apples, cubed and sprinkled with lemon juice
⅓ cup (75 ml) roasted hazelnuts, coarsely chopped
3 oz (100 g) chèvre (goat) cheese, crumbled or in pieces

Vinaigrette

3 tbsp (45 ml) extra virgin olive oil
2 tbsp (30 ml) lemon juice
1 tsp (5 ml) Dijon mustard

Instructions

- Grill hazelnuts (to dry out thoroughly) for 5 minutes in an oven at 350ºF (180ºC).
- Prepare vinaigrette by beating together oil, lemon juice and mustard.
- Arrange a mixture of the cubed apples, hazelnut and cheese on a bed of cress.
- Sprinkle with the vinaigrette, mix carefully and serve.

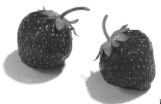

Strawberry Cantaloupe Avocado Salad

Served before a meal of grilled foods, this colorful salad nicely combines the antioxidant benefits of the strawberry with the softness of the avocado. It also stimulates the appetite and aids in digestion.

Ingredients *(4 servings)*

¾ cup (180 ml) small strawberries (or larger strawberries cut in halves or quarters)
1 medium cantaloupe, cut into bite-size pieces
1 ripe avocado, cut into bite-size pieces, drizzled with lemon juice
2 tbsp (30 ml) grapeseed or sunflower oil
2 tbsp (30 ml) hazelnut or peanut oil
1 tbsp (15 ml) apple cider vinegar
1 bunch fresh coriander leaves, chopped
1 cup (250 ml) mixed lettuce leaves (such as roquette, mesclun, spinach and cress), washed and dried
salt and pepper to taste

Instructions

- Line four dessert bowls with the salad leaves and fill with a mixture of the three fruits.
- Prepare vinaigrette by mixing the oils, apple cider vinegar, coriander, and salt and pepper to taste. Drizzle the fruit and salad greens with vinaigrette. Serve.

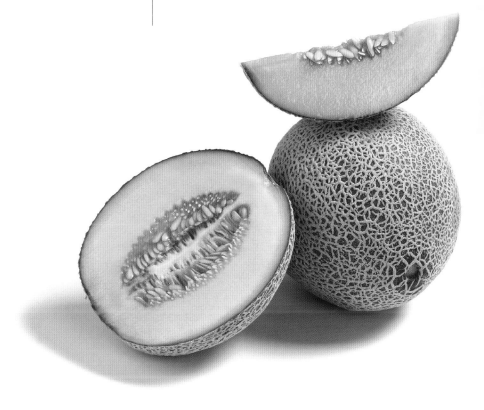

Papaya Shrimp Salad with Kiwi

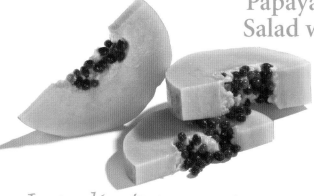

Inspired by a Thai recipe, this delicious appetizer can be prepared quickly. It is a fruit salad that beautifully combines two health-giving nutrients: the vitamin C of the papaya and the iron of the shrimp and spinach.

Ingredients *(4 servings)*

1 ripe papaya, seeded,* chopped into bite-size pieces
40 cooked shrimp, shelled
3 tbsp (45 ml) plain yogurt
3 tbsp (45 ml) light mayonnaise or tofu mayonnaise (see page 224)
¼ tsp (1 ml) red curry paste
2 bunches fresh coriander leaves, chopped
salt and pepper
2 ripe kiwis, peeled and sliced
spinach leaves and pitted black olives for garnish

* If you wish, you can wash, dry and grind the seeds from the papaya as a substitute for black pepper. It can then be sprinkled on this appetizer before serving.

Instructions

- Prepare sauce by mixing the yogurt, mayonnaise, curry paste and coriander leaves in a large bowl.
- Add shrimp and papaya pieces and mix carefully; cover with the yogurt-coriander mixture.
- Arrange kiwi slices and spinach leaves in four dessert cups. Add prepared papaya shrimp salad to each cup and garnish with black olives.

Variation

Omega-3-rich salmon version

Replace the shrimp with bite-size pieces of fresh salmon fillet, poached in the microwave (see page 198).

Tomato Salad with Fresh Basil

This simple, refreshing and delicious salad creates a happy marriage of several foods that offer excellent protection against cancer.

Ingredients *(4 servings)*

4 fully ripe tomatoes, sliced thinly
3 small cloves of garlic, minced
1 tsp (5 ml) lemon juice
2 tbsp (30 ml) extra virgin olive oil
2 tbsp (30 ml) fresh basil leaves, chopped
salt and pepper

Instructions

- Mix together the vinaigrette (garlic, lemon juice, olive oil and basil leaves) in a small bowl. Arrange the tomato slices in a single layer on a serving platter, and drizzle with vinaigrette.
- Season with salt and pepper and serve at once.

Buckwheat Vege-Pâté

This healthy substitute for pâté de foie gras is a light, highly nutritious appetizer you will want to serve to your dinner guests. Free of gluten, the dish is ideal for people who suffer from celiac disease (an allergy to the gluten in wheat and other grains).

Ingredients *(8 servings)*

1 cup (250 ml) unsalted sunflower seeds, ground
½ cup (125 ml) buckwheat flour
½ cup (125 ml) flakes of nutritional yeast (sold in health food stores)
1 onion, finely chopped
1 small zucchini, grated
1 carrot, grated
2 tbsp (30 ml) lemon juice
zest of ½ lemon
½ cup (125 ml) non-hydrogenated margarine
1 ½ cups (375 ml) boiling water
1 small clove of garlic, minced
1 tsp (5 ml) dried basil
salt and pepper

Instructions

- Preheat oven to 350ºF (180ºC).
- Mix together all the ingredients and pour into a loaf pan. Cook for 1 hour or until surface is lightly browned. Allow to cool, then chill in the refrigerator. Serve cold with whole grain bread, crackers or crisp breads.

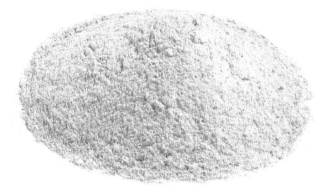

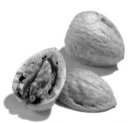

Walnut-Stuffed Tomatoes

Served before a meal containing starchy foods, this light appetizer will help with digestion and contains nutrients that protect against cancer. These delicious tomatoes also go wonderfully alongside a meat dish.

Ingredients *(4 servings)*

2 slices of toast, cut into small cubes
2 tbsp (30 ml) melted butter
2 tbsp (30 ml) chopped fresh basil or parsley
1 small clove of garlic, minced
3 tbsp (45 ml) shelled walnuts, chopped
2 tomatoes, cut in half, insides scooped out

Préparation

- Preheat oven to 375ºF (190ºC).
- Mix the bread cubes, melted butter, herbs, garlic and walnuts in a bowl.
- Fill the four tomato halves with the mixture.
- Bake for 10 minutes.

Chick-Pea Dip

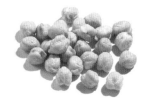

A delicious purée, inspired by a Middle Eastern recipe, this dip supplies an excellent amount of dietary fiber and protects against cardiovascular disease.

Ingredients *(8 servings)*

19-oz (540-ml) can of chick-peas, drained and rinsed
1 clove of garlic, minced
1 tbsp (15 ml) lemon juice
zest of ½ lemon
1 tbsp (15 ml) olive oil
a few drops chili sauce or Harissa Chili Sauce (see page 223), to taste
2 tbsp (30 ml) tahini*
½ tsp (2 ml) ground cumin
2 tbsp (30 ml) fresh coriander, chopped

* Tahini is a purée made from sesame seeds, found in many specialty and health food shops.

Instructions

- In a blender or food processor, mix the chick-peas to a paste.
- Add garlic, lemon juice and zest, olive oil, chili sauce, tahini and cumin. Process together until smooth.
- Garnish with the chopped coriander and serve with bread, wedges of pita bread or crackers.

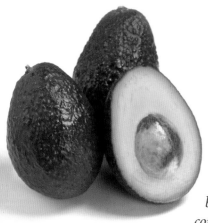

Avocado Dip with Lemon and Anchovy

Offering a delicate combination of flavors, this appetizer is rich in beneficial omega-3 fatty acids and goes especially well before a main course of fish.

Instructions

- In a bowl, mash the avocado with a fork.
- Add anchovy, lemon juice and zest, and mix well.
- Serve as a dip for fresh raw vegetables or as a spread on crackers.

Ingredients *(4 servings)*

1 ripe avocado, peeled and pitted
4 small anchovy fillets, finely chopped
1 tsp (5 ml) lemon juice and the zest of ½ lemon

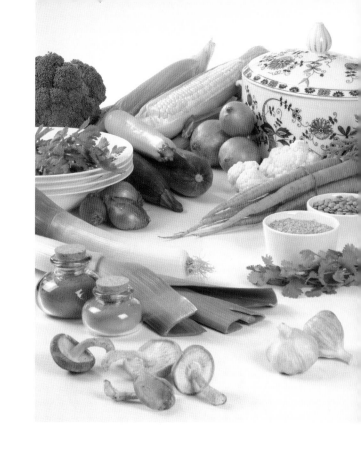

Soups

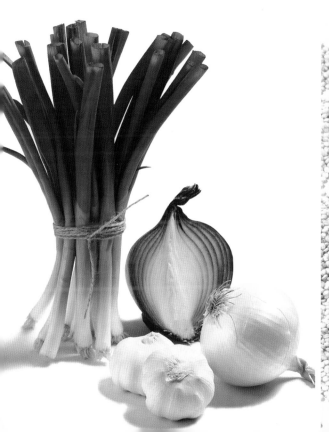

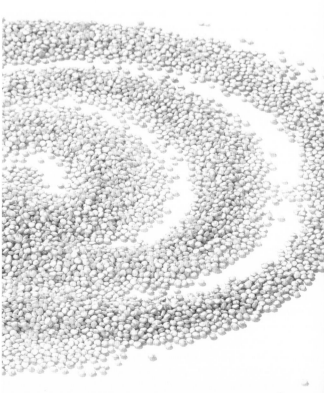

The Secret To Great Soups

Believe it or not, along with salads, soups are the food that provides us with the most health-giving nutrients for our bodies. How is this possible? Well, both of these foods allow us to include in our diet the widest variety of vegetables, grains, pulses, herbs and spices. And as you have seen in Part One, the key to benefiting most from the potent, natural medicinal properties of foods is to increase the variety of healing foods in your diet.

For hundreds—if not thousands—of years, soups have always been a convenience food, using ingredients readily at hand to make life simpler. And for the more clumsy cooks among us, soups are practically impossible to ruin. The only rule of thumb to keep in mind is that you should always begin with a good homemade soup broth. Chicken or beef bouillon, which is simply a filtered broth, is a natural remedy that our grandmothers and great-grandmothers recommended for protecting the body against colds, for calming upset stomachs, or for restoring and fortifying the body after an illness. To this day, soup broth or bouillon can provide us with a whole host of proven benefits.

The Homemade Chicken Broth and Homemade Vegetable Broth recipes included on the following pages take very little time to prepare and are well worth the extra bit of planning required. The chicken broth also makes efficient use of the bones and carcass once you've enjoyed a delicious dinner of roast chicken. After the broth is made, simply toss in whatever vegetables you choose (or whatever is close to hand) to create soups that, depending on their consistency, can be served either at the beginning of a meal or as a hearty main course 'comfort food'.

Soup Recipes

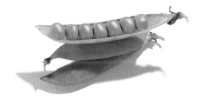

Homemade Chicken Broth

This broth is full of flavors and costs almost nothing to make since it is prepared with the carcass of a chicken or turkey that would otherwise be thrown away once the best bits of meat have been removed. This excellent broth can also be used for delicious gravies and sauces, as well as quick lunchtime soups.

Ingredients

1 carcass of a roast chicken, turkey, duck, etc. (that is, the cooking juices or drippings, the skin and bones including the neck, the heart and kidneys, but not the liver)
1 onion, whole, peeled
1 carrot, whole, scrubbed but not peeled
1 celery stalk, leaves included
1 clove of garlic, peeled
1 piece of fresh ginger, peeled
1 bunch of parsley
1 bay leaf
1 tsp (5 ml) dried mixed herbs (thyme, basil, oregano, chervil)
salt and pepper to taste

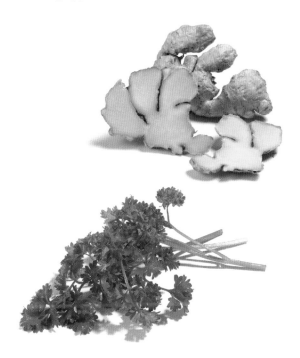

Instruction

- Place poultry carcass, juices and organs in a large pot.
- Add all remaining ingredients and enough cold water to cover carcass (about 3 quarts, or 3 liters).
- Bring to a boil, season to taste, reduce heat and leave to simmer, covered, for at least 2 hours.
- Allow to cool for several hours (or overnight if making in the evening), then filter through a colander or sieve. Broth will keep for several days in the refrigerator, covered with its own grease. To use, simply skim off grease. Once de-greased and frozen, broth will keep for up to six months.

Variation

Different poultry broths

As mentioned, a flavorful broth can be prepared with the carcass of other types of poultry, such as turkey, duck, pheasant, goose, quail or guinea hen.

Suggestion

A quick lunchtime soup

Using the homemade broth, this quick soup is a wonderful pick-me-up, especially on a cold day. Simply add a few teaspoons of couscous, sliced mushroom, parsley, thinly sliced carrot and spicy salsa, and you will have a delicious, hearty soup within five minutes.

Homemade Vegetable Broth

This soup broth contains a bevy of healthy nutrients that will enrich all of your soups and stews. For a touch of something exotic, replace the traditional herb mixture (thyme, basil, oregano, chervil) with a mixture of cumin, fennel seed, curry, chili powder, star anise and coriander.

Ingredients

2 onions, whole, peeled (or 2 leeks)
2 carrots, scrubbed, unpeeled
1 parsnip, scrubbed
4 celery stalks, leaves included
1 clove of garlic
3 quarts (3 liters) water
2 bay leaves
1 tbsp (15 ml) mixed herbs (e.g. thyme, basil, oregano, chervil)
salt and pepper to taste

Instructions

- Place all vegetables in a large pot and cover with water.
- Bring to a boil, reduce heat and leave to simmer, covered, for at least 1 hour.
- Let cool, then filter through a colander or sieve. Discard or compost the vegetables. Store broth in the refrigerator.

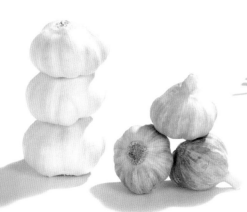

Creamy Garlic and Vegetable Soup

Naturally fortifying, this soup is a great comfort food that helps to protect against early cold symptoms… or to fight a full-blown virus!

Ingredients

6 cups (1.5 liters) Homemade Chicken Broth (see page 165)
1 whole bulb of garlic, cloves peeled and minced
4 medium carrots, washed (unpeeled), chopped into pieces
1 small rutabaga, cut into cubes
4 small zucchinis, peeled and cut into pieces
¼ cup (60 ml) fresh parsley, chopped
salt and pepper to taste

Instructions

- Place all the ingredients, except for the parsley, salt and pepper, into a large 2-quart (2-liter) soup pot.
- Bring to a boil, reduce heat slightly and simmer for 20 minutes or until vegetables are cooked.
- Let cool, then put in a blender and mix to a smooth consistency.
- Reheat, season to taste, add parsley and serve.

Butternut Squash Soup

Perfumed with curry, this rich winter soup is full of beta carotene from the squash. Beta carotene, an antioxidant, offers protection against colds and infections.

Ingredients *(4 servings)*

1 onion, chopped
2 shallots, minced
3 tbsp (45 ml) olive oil
1 clove of garlic, minced
1 tsp (5 ml) curry powder
1 butternut* squash, peeled, seeded and cubed
2 medium carrots, chopped
2 ½ cups (625 ml) Homemade Vegetable Broth or Homemade Chicken Broth (see pages 166 and 165)
½ cup (125 ml) unsweetened evaporated milk, unflavored soy drink or coconut milk (optional)
salt and pepper to taste

Instruction

- Heat olive oil in a large saucepan and sauté the onion and shallot without browning.
- Add garlic, curry powder, squash, carrots and broth.
- Bring to a boil, lower the heat and simmer for 25 minutes.
- Let cool, then transfer to a blender and mix to uniform consistency.
- Season with salt and pepper. If the soup is still too thick, thin with evaporated milk, soy drink or coconut milk.

* Butternut squash is so called because of its rich buttery flavor.

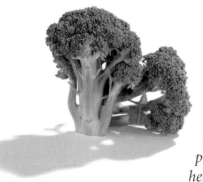

Broccoli Soup

This soup features broccoli, a vegetable with an astonishing number of health-giving nutrients, including glucoraphanin, a powerful antioxidant that protects against cardiovascular disease and helps prevent various forms of cancer.

Ingredients *(4 to 6 servings)*

2 tbsp (30 ml) olive oil
1 onion, chopped (or 1 leek, sliced)
2 medium potatoes, chopped
3 stems of broccoli, separated into florets
2 cloves of garlic, minced
4 cups (1 litre) Homemade Chicken Broth (see page 165)
salt and pepper to taste

Instructions

- In a large pot, sauté onion or leek lightly in the oil without browning.
- Add all of the remaining ingredients and bring to a boil.
- Lower the heat to medium and let simmer for 20 minutes.
- Let cool, then mix to a smooth consistency in a blender. Reheat to serve.

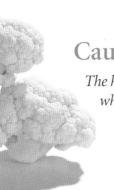

Cauliflower Soup

The high fiber content of cauliflower helps to neutralize certain fats when this soup is served before a main course of meat.

Ingredients *(4 to 6 servings)*

2 tbsp (30 ml) olive oil
1 onion, chopped
1 head of cauliflower, separated into florets
3 medium potatoes, peeled and cut into quarters
2 zucchinis, peeled and cut into pieces
1 clove of garlic, minced
4 cups (1 liter) Homemade Chicken Broth
(see page 165)
2 tbsp (30 ml) fresh herbs (basil, parsley or
coriander)
salt and pepper to taste

Instructions

- In a large pot, sauté onion lightly in the oil without browning.
- Add the cauliflower florets, potato and zucchini, and cook for a few minutes.
- Add the garlic and chicken broth and bring to a boil.
- Lower the heat to medium and let simmer for 20 minutes.
- Let cool, then mix to a smooth consistency in a blender.
- Add the herbs and mix again.
- Season to taste and reheat before serving.

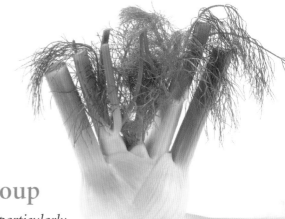

Fennel Soup

This soup has an aroma of aniseed from the fennel. It is particularly beneficial for people with intestinal afflictions or gas.

Ingredients *(4 to 6 servings)*

2 tbsp (30 ml) olive oil
1 shallot, chopped
1 whole fennel bulb, sliced into strips
2 large zucchinis (or 3 small), unpeeled, cut into
pieces
1 clove of garlic, minced
3 cups (750 ml) Homemade Chicken Broth
(see page 165)
salt and pepper to taste

Instructions

- In a large pot, sauté the shallot in the oil without browning.
- Add fennel and zucchini and cook for a few minutes over low heat.
- Add garlic and chicken broth and bring to a boil.
- Lower the heat and let simmer for 20 minutes.
- Let cool, then mix to a smooth consistency in a blender.
- Return soup to the heat, season to taste, and serve.

Parsnip and Zucchini Soup

Parsnips bring a delectable flavor to this soup, making it particularly heart-warming. Low in calories, this uniquely flavored vegetable offers prevention against cardiovascular disease.

Ingredients *(6 to 8 servings)*

2 tbsp (30 ml) olive oil
2 onions, chopped
3 parsnips (leaves removed) washed, brushed and cubed
2 zucchinis, unpeeled, cut into pieces
1 potato, unpeeled, cut into pieces
1 clove of garlic, minced
6 cups (1.5 liters) Homemade Chicken Broth (see page 165)
salt and pepper to taste

Instructions

- In a large pot, sauté the onions in the oil without browning.
- Add all of the remaining ingredients and bring to a boil.
- Lower the heat and let simmer for 20 minutes.
- Let cool, then mix to a smooth consistency in a blender.
- Season to taste and serve hot.

Mushroom Soup

The subtle flavor of the shiitake mushrooms, with their renowned anti-viral properties, will easily direct your attention away from the earthy-brown color of this soup. If you do want to improve its appearance, add a few chopped leaves of spinach just a minute or two before removing the soup from the stove.

Ingredients *(4 servings)*

2 shallots, chopped
2 tbsp (30 ml) non-hydrogenated margarine
3.5-oz (100-g) packet of fresh shiitake mushrooms,* sliced
8-oz (227-g) package of fresh white button mushrooms, sliced
3 zucchinis, peeled and cut into pieces
1 clove of garlic, minced
3 cups (750 ml) Homemade Chicken Broth (see page 165)
a few spinach leaves
salt and pepper to taste

Préparation

- In a large pot, sauté the shallots in the margarine without browning.
- Add the mushrooms and zucchini and cook for a few minutes, stirring constantly.
- Add garlic and broth and bring to a boil.
- Lower the heat and let simmer, covered, for 20 minutes.
- Let cool, then mix to a smooth consistency in a blender.
- Season to taste and serve hot.

* If using dried mushrooms, re-hydrate in a little warm water, then drain and cut off the stems before adding to the soup mixture.

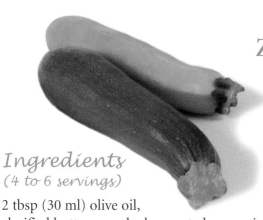

Zucchini Soup

Low in calories and with a sensational flavour, this soup has a simplicity that will delight anyone.

Ingredients
(4 to 6 servings)

2 tbsp (30 ml) olive oil,
clarified butter or unhydrogenated margarine
1 shallot, chopped
5 or 6 medium zucchinis, unpeeled, cut into pieces
2 cloves of garlic, minced
4 cups (1 liter) Homemade Chicken Broth (see page 165)
salt and pepper to taste

Instructions

- In a large pot, sauté the shallot in the oil, butter or margarine, without browning.
- Add zucchini and cook for a few minutes.
- Add garlic and broth and bring to a boil.
- Lower the heat and let simmer for 20 minutes.
- Let cool, then mix to a smooth consistency in a blender.
- Season to taste and serve hot.

Spinach Soup with Pecans

This hearty winter soup is a whole meal in itself. Comprised of two ingredients not often found together in a soup, the spinach and pecans are a delicious combination of fortifying, anti-viral properties.

Ingredients *(6 servings)*

6 cups (1.5 liters) Homemade Chicken Broth (see page 165)
2 oz. (60 g) fine noodles
2 cups (500 ml) spinach leaves, washed and chopped
½ cup (125 ml) fresh parsley, chopped
½ cup (125 ml) fresh basil leaves, chopped
¼ cup (60 ml) pecans, coarsely chopped
1 clove of garlic, minced
2 tbsp (30 ml) olive oil
salt and pepper to taste

Instructions

- Bring to a boil 5 cups (1.25 liters) of the chicken broth in a large pot. Add noodles and cook until *al dente*.
- Meanwhile, use a blender to purée together the spinach, the remaining 1 cup (250 ml) of broth and the parsley. Add basil, pecans and garlic. Mix together in a blender for one minute more. Add the oil.
- Mix the spinach-pecan mixture with the noodles. Heat.
- Season to taste and serve hot.

Curried Celery Soup

Savory and full of seasoning, this soup has the benefit of reuniting all parts of the celery plant, thereby offering a soup with excellent digestive qualities.

Ingredients *(4 servings)*

2 tbsp (30 ml) olive oil
1 onion, chopped
1 shallot, chopped
6 stalks of celery, sliced
2 medium potatoes, peeled and diced
1 tsp (5 ml) curry powder
3 cups (750 ml) Homemade Chicken Broth or Homemade Vegetable Broth (see pages 165 and 166)
2 tbsp (30 ml) fresh herbs for aroma (basil, tarragon or coriander)
celery seeds and leaves
salt and pepper to taste

Instructions

- In a large pot, sauté the onion, shallot and celery in the oil for a few minutes without browning.
- Add all other ingredients except for the herbs, celery seeds and leaves. Bring to a boil.
- Lower the heat and let simmer for 20 minutes.
- Allow to cool. Mix to a smooth consistency in a blender.
- Season to taste, add the fresh herbs and mix again.
- Return to heat. Decorate serving dishes with celery leaves and seeds. Serve the soup hot.

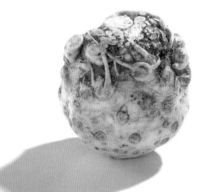

Sweet Potato and Celeriac Soup

This warming soup is a great cold-fighter and has a refined flavor—the result of combining two vegetables packed with vitamins.

Ingredients *(4 servings)*

1 whole root of celeriac, peeled and diced
1 sweet potato, peeled and diced
1 leek (or 1 onion), finely chopped
1 zucchini, peeled and cut into pieces
1 tbsp (15 ml) olive oil
3 cups (750 ml) water, Homemade Chicken Broth or Homemade Vegetable Broth (see pages 165 and 166)
1 bunch of fresh coriander, finely chopped

Instructions

- Sauté the vegetables in the oil for 1 minute in a large pot.
- Add the water or broth and bring to a boil.
- Lower the heat and allow to simmer, covered, for 20 minutes.
- Season to taste and leave to cool.
- Mix to a smooth consistency in a blender. Serve hot, garnished with coriander.

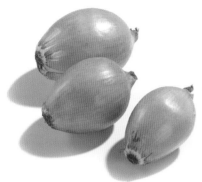

Onion Soup with Dulse

Onion soup is a great pick-me-up for the day after a big feast, and it is a cleansing remedy for indigestion. The soup also offers good protection against colds and viruses.

Ingredients *(4 servings)*

4 large onions, peeled, sliced into fine rings
2 shallots, chopped
2 tbsp (30 ml) clarified butter (see instructions on page 152)
1 tbsp (15 ml) olive oil
3 cups (750 ml) unsalted beef bouillon or Homemade Chicken Broth (see page 165)
1 tbsp (15 ml) flakes of dulse
2 cloves of garlic, minced
2 bay leaves
pepper to taste

Instructions

- In a large pot, sauté the shallot and onion in the butter and oil, without browning.
- Add the broth, dulse flakes, garlic and bay leaves. Bring to a boil.
- Lower the heat and let simmer for 20 minutes.
- Season with pepper and serve with fresh, crusty bread or crackers.

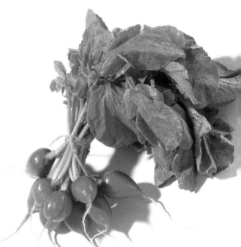

Radish-Leaf Soup

This soup, like the onion soup above, is a great comfort food with anti-viral properties. It is also a great way to make use of radish leaves after using the radishes themselves in a salad.

Ingredients *(6 to 8 servings)*

2 tbsp (30 ml) olive oil
2 leeks, finely chopped
1 bunch fresh radish leaves, washed and chopped
4 potatoes, peeled and diced
5 cups (1.25 liters) water or Homemade Vegetable Broth (see page 166)
1 pinch of nutmeg
½ cup (125 ml) milk or soy milk
salt and pepper to taste

Instructions

- In a large pot, sauté the leek in the oil without browning.
- Add radish leaves and cook, covered, at low heat for a few minutes.
- Add potatoes, water or broth, nutmeg and seasoning. Bring to a boil.
- Lower the heat and let simmer for 20 minutes.
- Leave to cool. Mix to a smooth consistency in a blender.
- Return to soup pot, add the milk or soy drink and serve hot.

Lentil Soup

This wonderful soup is very rich in dietary fiber and is especially beneficial for people who are struggling with high levels of "bad" (LDL) cholesterol.

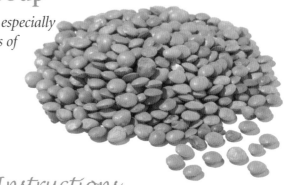

Ingredients *(8 servings)*

1 tbsp (15 ml) olive oil
2 cloves of garlic, minced
2 onions, chopped
1 stalk of celery, chopped
3 carrots, diced
1 tsp (5 ml) curry powder
6 cups (1.5 liters) Homemade Chicken Broth or Homemade Vegetable Broth (see pages 165 and 166)
1 tbsp (15 ml) tomato paste
1 cup (250 ml) red or green lentils, rinsed
1 to 2 cups (250 to 500 ml) spinach leaves, washed and chopped
salt and pepper to taste

Instructions

- Sauté garlic and onion in the oil in a large pot.
- Add celery, carrots, curry powder, broth and tomato paste, and bring to a boil.
- Lower the heat and let simmer for 10 minutes.
- Add lentils and cook for another 10 minutes.
- Add spinach and simmer for 5 more minutes before serving.

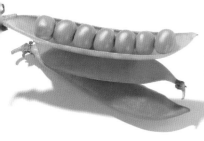

Fresh Green Pea Soup

This flavorful soup, which is just as fine in the summer as in winter, contains an abundance of vitamins and other compounds that help protect the body against cardiovascular disease.

Ingredients *(6 servings)*

2 tbsp (30 ml) olive oil
2 large onions, finely chopped
1 stalk of celery, chopped
1 medium zucchini, peeled and cut into pieces
1 clove of garlic, minced
1 tsp (5 ml) curry powder
1 tsp (5 ml) turmeric
4 cups (1 liter) Homemade Chicken broth or Homemade Vegetable Broth (see pages 165 and 166)
2 cups (500 ml) frozen peas
salt and pepper to taste

Instruction

- In a large pot, sauté the onion in the oil without browning.
- Add celery, zucchini, garlic, spices and half of the broth.
- Bring to a boil. Cover and let simmer on low heat for 20 minutes.
- Add the peas and remaining broth. Bring to a boil.
- Lower the heat again and simmer for 10 more minutes.
- Let cool, season to taste, then mix to a smooth consistency in a blender.
- Serve hot.

Indian Split Pea Soup

Deliciously scented, this low-calorie soup is rich in dietary fiber and minerals, and helps to combat anemia.

Ingredients *(6 to 8 servings)*

1 leek, white part only, minced
1 carrot, washed and cubed
2 tbsp (30 ml) olive oil
½ tsp (2 ml) each of the following spices:
cinnamon, cumin, ground ginger, ground black
pepper, turmeric, fenugreek
1 pinch of cloves
2 cloves of garlic, minced
6 cups (1.5 liters) water or Homemade Vegetable
Broth (see page 166)
1 cup (250 ml) split peas, washed and drained
12 spinach leaves, well washed
salt and pepper to taste

Instructions

- In a large pot, sauté the leek and carrot in the oil without browning.
- Add the spices and cook for another minute on low heat.
- Add garlic, water or broth, and split peas, and bring to a boil.
- Lower the heat and let simmer, covered, for about 35 minutes or until the peas are tender.
- Add the spinach and season to taste. Turn up the heat and simmer for another 5 minutes before serving.

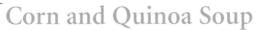

Corn and Quinoa Soup

This well-seasoned soup combines two ingredients cherished by South Americans: corn and quinoa. The latter is renowned for its regenerative and fortifying properties.

Instructions

- In a large pot, sauté the onion in the oil without browning.
- Add the sweet pepper and corn. Cook, covered, for 10 minutes.
- Add the broth and Harissa Sauce and bring to a boil. Reduce heat and let simmer for another 10 minutes.
- Add quinoa, season with salt and pepper and continue cooking for 10 minutes before serving.

Ingredients *(6 servings)*

2 tbsp (30 ml) grapeseed oil
1 onion, minced
1 sweet red pepper, cubed
1 ½ cups (375 ml) fresh corn kernels, or one
12-oz (340-ml) can of kernel corn
4 cups (1 liter) Homemade Chicken Broth (see
page 165)
1 tsp (5 ml) Harissa Chili Sauce (see page 223)
4 tbsp (60 ml) quinoa, carefully rinsed
salt and pepper to taste

Variation

For a soup rich in calcium, leave out the red pepper and replace 1 cup (250 ml) of the broth with 1 cup (250 ml) of plain soy drink. Cool and process in a blender. Reheat soup and garnish with chopped coriander or parsley before serving.

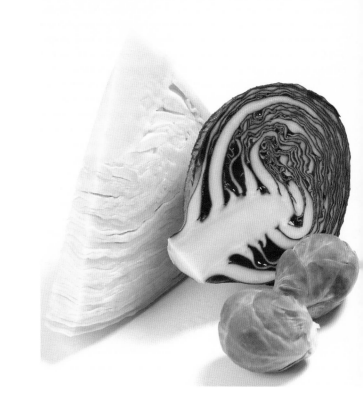

Side Dishes

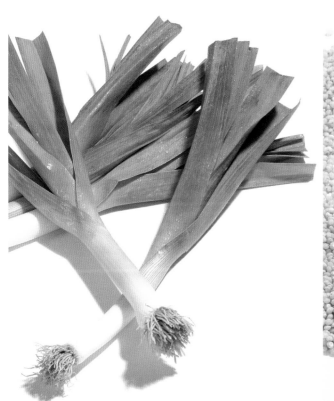

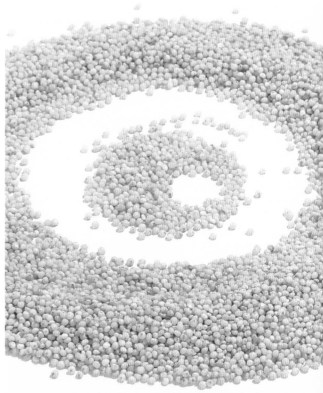

Side Dishes:
Partners in Health

To accompany a main course, a side dish must both contrast and enhance its flavors. It must also be somewhat low-key, so as not to dominate the overall taste experience. A well-chosen side dish is one that rebalances the meal; for example, it should counter the sometimes overly rich fats of the meat dish in a main course. Vegetables are the best foods to play this role, especially in a meal with meat, since they will counteract greasy fats with their high-fiber, vitamin-rich content.

If you consume several servings of meat in a single week, be sure to accompany your main dishes with substantial portions of vegetables. Consult the following pages to try side dishes that are new and different, and to add more variety to your meals. Rice and other grains in a side dish offer a very healthy combination for people who do not generally eat as much at mealtimes, or for people who are lacking the health-giving virtues that grains offer.

Side Dish Recipes

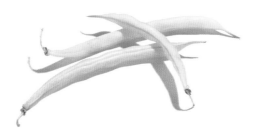

Indian-Style
Braised Cauliflower

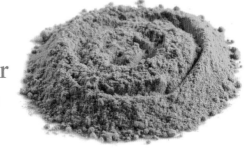

Thanks to the rich aromas of the spices and broth, this plain vegetable is transformed into a delicious side dish full of fortifying vitamins and health-giving dietary fiber.

Ingredients *(4 to 6 servings)*

1 head of cauliflower
3 tbsp (45 ml) clarified butter (see page 152) or non-hydrogenated margarine
1 tsp (5 ml) fresh ginger, grated
½ tsp (2 ml) turmeric
1 tsp (5 ml) cumin seeds
1 cup (250 ml) Homemade Chicken Broth (see page 165)
1 ½ tbsp (22 ml) clarified butter (see page 152)
1 ½ tbsp (22 ml) flour
salt and pepper to taste

Instructions

- Break up cauliflower into small florets.
- Soak cauliflower for 1 hour in cold water to remove bitterness, then drain carefully.
- Melt 3 tbsp (45 ml) butter or margarine in a large pot.
- Add ginger and turmeric and sauté over low heat for 30 seconds.
- Add cauliflower and mix well so that the florets become coated in spices.
- Add salt, pepper and cumin.
- Stir in broth, cover and bring to a boil.
- Lower the heat and cook for 15 minutes.
- While the cauliflower is still crunchy, prepare the sauce by mixing together 1 ½ tbsp (22 ml) clarified butter and the flour over low heat in a small saucepan.
- Remove the cauliflower from the broth and set aside. Pour the broth into the flour-butter mixture and heat until sauce thickens.
- Top the cauliflower with the sauce and serve.

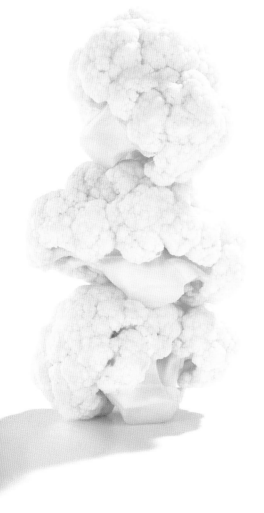

Sautéed Brussels Sprouts

Here is a simple and delicious way to make use of these vegetables that contain potent, well-known anti-viral properties.

Ingredients *(4 servings)*

2 cups (500 ml) Brussels sprouts (wilted leaves removed), washed
2 tbsp (30 ml) olive oil or clarified butter (see page 152)
6 green onions or 2 shallots, minced
½ sweet red pepper, diced
1 clove of garlic, minced
1 tbsp (15 ml) soy sauce or tamari
zest and juice of ½ lemon
2 tbsp (30 ml) sesame seeds
salt and pepper to taste

Instructions

- Soak Brussels sprouts for 30 minutes in a bowl of water with 1 tsp (5 ml) of vinegar added.
- In a saucepan, sauté the green onions or shallots and red pepper in the oil without browning.
- Add the Brussels sprouts, garlic, soy sauce, ¼ cup (60 ml) water and lemon juice, and bring to a boil.
- Cover, lower the heat and let simmer for 10 minutes.
- Adjust seasoning, garnish with lemon zest and sesame seeds. Serve warm.

Braised Endives

The lemon juice in this dish counterbalances the bitterness of the endives and gives a delicious flavor. These low-calorie vegetables are especially recommended for pregnant women and nursing mothers.

Instructions

- Put endives in a saucepan with ½ cup (125 ml) water and the sugar.
- Bring to a boil and remove from the heat as soon as the water boils.
- Discard the sugar water. Set aside endives.
- Melt butter in the saucepan and braise the endives for 10 minutes over low heat, or until they are tender and slightly caramelized, making sure they do not burn.
- Sprinkle with lemon juice and serve alongside a grilled main dish.

Ingredients *(2 servings)*

4 very fresh endives
1 tsp (5 ml) sugar
1 tbsp (15 ml) butter
2 tbsp (30 ml) lemon juice

Braised Fennel in Tomato Sauce

Cooked in a tomato sauce, this fennel dish makes for a delectable appetizer that also helps to combat intestinal gas.

Ingredients *(4 servings)*

1 whole fennel bulb, fronds trimmed

1 tbsp (15 ml) olive oil

¼ cup (60 ml) white wine

1 cup (250 ml) Fresh Tomato Sauce (see page 226)

10 or 12 Kalamata black olives, pitted and chopped

½ cup (125 ml) breadcrumbs mixed with chopped nuts or grated cheese (depending on whether the dish is to be served as an appetizer or side dish), for topping

Instructions

- Preheat oven to 350ºF (180ºC).
- Cut the fennel in quarters lengthwise and remove the tough part at the center.
- In a large pot, heat the oil and sauté the fennel. Add the white wine, cover and cook over very low heat for about 20 minutes (making sure the fennel does not caramelize) until just *al dente*.
- Arrange fennel in a baking dish. Pour over the tomato sauce and olive pieces.
- Bake for 20 minutes until cooked *au gratin*, or golden brown.

Variation

- Replace the tomato sauce with a meat sauce to make a delicious main course for two.

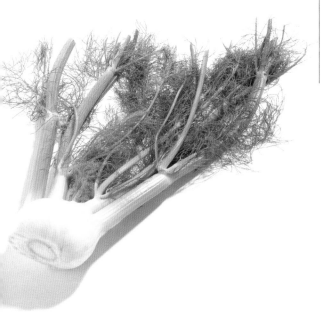

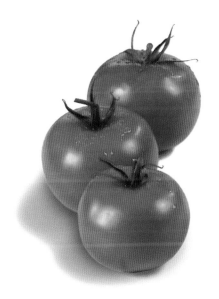

Fresh Beans with Capers and Lemon

This tasty side dish is recommended for people suffering from anemia or for those who are convalescing after a hospital stay or illness.

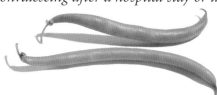

Ingredients *(4 servings)*

1 lb (500 g) fresh beans, washed and trimmed
2 tbsp (30 ml) olive oil
1 small shallot, minced
2 tbsp (30 ml) capers
1 tsp (5 ml) lemon juice
zest of ½ lemon
fresh basil leaves, chopped, for garnish

Instructions

- Steam the beans for 15 minutes or until *al dente*.
- Five minutes before the beans are cooked, heat oil in a saucepan and sauté the shallot over medium heat without browning.
- Add capers and lemon juice, then add the steamed beans.
- Add the lemon zest, season to taste and decorate with fresh basil. Serve.

Millet Casserole

Millet is a grain rich in niacin, a vitamin that helps slow the decline of the mental faculties and may reduce the risk of Alzheimer's disease.

Ingredients *(4 servings)*

1 cup (250 ml) wholegrain millet
2 ¼ cups (560 ml) cold water
3 tbsp (45 ml) olive oil
2 onions, minced
2 carrots, diced
¼ cup (60 ml) celery leaves, chopped
2 cloves of garlic, minced
¼ tsp (1 ml) thyme
salt and pepper to taste
grated Gruyère cheese

Instructions

- Rinse the millet, cover with cold water and leave to soak for 2 hours.
- Heat the oil and sauté vegetables and seasonings for a few minutes.
- Add the millet with its soaking water. Bring to a boil.
- Lower the heat and let simmer, covered, for 25 minutes or until the millet is tender.
- Transfer to a baking dish, sprinkle with the grated cheese and cook at 375ºF (190ºC) until it is *au gratin*, or golden brown (about 10 minutes).

Plantains with Parsnip and Coriander

Plantain is believed by many to help relieve stomach ulcers and different types of inflammation. Add variety to your diet by replacing baked potato with this dish; it goes very well with grilled meats.

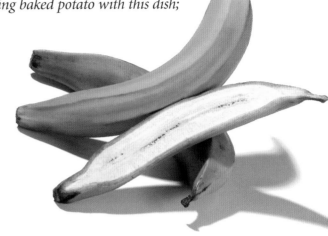

Ingredients *(4 servings)*

1 tbsp (15 ml) olive oil
2 shallots, minced
1 clove of garlic, minced
2 plantains, peeled and diced
1 medium-sized parsnip, diced
½ cup (125 ml) Homemade Chicken Broth (see page 165)
1 bunch of fresh coriander (cilantro) leaves, chopped
salt and pepper to taste

Instructions

- In a large pot, sauté the shallots in the oil without browning.
- Add garlic, plantain, parsnip and broth. Bring to a boil.
- Lower the heat and let simmer, covered, for 20 minutes over low heat, making sure the parsnip does not brown.
- Add coriander and serve.

Jerusalem Artichoke and Mushrooms

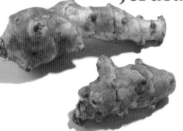

People suffering from hypertension will benefit from the subtle flavor of the Jerusalem artichoke in this dish—a flavor that tastes of both hazelnuts and artichoke and blends very well with the mushrooms. This wonderfully simple dish is perfect alongside grilled fish.

Instructions

- Put the Jerusalem artichokes into a pot of salted boiling water and cook for 20 minutes until just tender.
- Drain and let cool.
- Dice the Jerusalem artichokes, then sprinkle with lemon juice. Set aside.
- In a saucepan, melt the butter or margarine and sauté the shallot and garlic without browning.
- Add the mushrooms and Jerusalem artichoke, and cook for 5 to 10 minutes on low heat.
- Add the chopped herbs and serve immediately.

Ingredients *(4 servings)*

4 Jerusalem artichokes, washed and scrubbed
1 tbsp (15 ml) lemon juice
2 tbsp (30 ml) butter or non-hydrogenated margarine
1 shallot, chopped
1 clove of garlic, minced
8 oz (227 g) small white mushrooms, sliced
2 tbsp (30 ml) minced fresh parsley, chives, basil or other fresh herbs

Mashed Potatoes with Carrot and Rutabaga

This delicious purée of three nutritious root vegetables offers excellent protection against diseases of the liver.

Ingredients *(4 servings)*

3 large potatoes with yellow flesh (e.g. Yukon gold), peeled and cut into quarters
2 carrots, scrubbed, unpeeled and cut into pieces
1 rutabaga, cut into cubes
¼ cup (60 ml) fresh chives or parsley, chopped
1 tbsp (15 ml) butter or non-hydrogenated margarine

Instructions

- Boil the vegetables in a pot of salted water for 20 minutes.
- Drain and mash into a purée. Add the chives or parsley, then the butter or margarine to enrich the texture.
- Serve with meat, roast or grilled.

Tip

- This dish will keep for three days in the refrigerator. Refrigerate leftovers in single-serving, microwave-safe dishes or ramekins and reheat for 30 seconds in the microwave as needed.

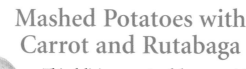

Curried Rice with Pistachio

The rice in this easily digested dish contains soluble fiber that helps to lower the risk of heart disease and several types of cancer. The Indian seasonings makes this an elegant side dish for grilled salmon sprinkled with lemon juice.

Ingredients *(4 to 6 servings)*

2 tbsp (30 ml) clarified butter (see page 152)
1 small onion, chopped
½ tsp (2 ml) of each of the following spices: turmeric, cardamom, crushed chili, coriander
1 tsp (5 ml) ground cumin
1 cup (250 ml) basmati, jasmine or other long-grain rice
2 cloves of garlic, minced
2 cups (500 ml) water, Homemade Chicken Broth or Homemade Vegetable Broth (see pages 165 or 166)
⅓ cup (75 ml) pistachios, shelled
salt and pepper to taste

Instructions

- In a large pot, sauté the onion in the clarified butter without browning.
- Add the spices and mix well. Cook for 2 minutes over low heat.
- Add rice and mix thoroughly to coat the grains in the spices.
- Add garlic and water or broth, and bring to a boil.
- Lower the heat and let simmer until the rice is cooked (15 to 25 minutes depending on the type of rice used).
- Taste, adjust seasoning and add the pistachios just before serving.

Rice with Leek, Mushroom and Fine Herbs

This deliciously seasoned rice dish with lemon is highly recommended for people with hypertension (high blood pressure). It is lovely alongside a main course of pan-fried fish fillets.

Ingredients *(4 to 6 servings)*

1 tbsp (15 ml) olive oil
1 small shallot, minced
1 cup (250 ml) long-grain rice
2 ¼ cups (560 ml) Homemade Chicken Broth (see page 165)
2 cloves of garlic, minced
1 tbsp (15 ml) olive oil
2 leeks, finely minced
1 tsp (5 ml) herbs Provençal (marjoram, thyme, basil, rosemary, savory)
1 cup (250 ml) sliced white mushrooms
grated zest of 1 lemon
salt and pepper to taste

Instructions

- In a large pot, sauté the shallot in 1 tsp (15 ml) olive oil without browning.
- Add rice, broth and garlic and bring to a boil.
- Lower the heat and let simmer for 20 minutes.
- Meanwhile, sauté the leeks in 1 tsp (15 ml) olive oil in a saucepan. Add the herbs and mushrooms and cook for 10 minutes over low heat.
- Once the rice has cooked (approximately 20 minutes), add the lemon zest followed by the leek-mushroom mixture.
- Mix well, season to taste and serve.

Brown Rice with Almond and Raisin

This rice dish is good for helping to lower high blood pressure. To serve it as a main course, simply add a choice of cooked vegetables (zucchini, broccoli, carrots, etc.) five minutes before the end of the cooking time, and increase the amount of raisins and almonds.

Ingredients *(4 servings)*

1 cup (250 ml) long-grain brown rice
1 tbsp (15 ml) clarified butter (see page 152) or olive oil
1 tsp (5 ml) herbs Provençal (marjoram, thyme, basil, rosemary, savory)
1 tsp (5 ml) orange zest, grated
2 ¼ cups (560 ml) Homemade Vegetable Broth (see page 166)
2 tbsp (30 ml) flaked almonds, toasted
2 tbsp (30 ml) raisins
salt and pepper to taste

Instructions

- Sauté the rice gently in the clarified butter or oil, coating it well.
- Add the herbs and orange zest and cook for 1 minute, stirring constantly.
- Add vegetable broth and bring to a boil.
- Cover, reduce heat and let simmer gently, without stirring, for about 25 minutes or until the liquid has been absorbed and the rice is tender.
- Remove from heat and add almonds and raisins.
- Correct the seasoning and let sit for 5 minutes before serving.

Indian-Style Rice and Sweet Potato Pie

This delicious, hearty, curry-seasoned pie is rich in dietary fiber and vitamins. It can be served as an appetizer or as a side dish with a main course. Because it is rich and filling without being high in calories, it is especially good for diabetics and for people who are watching their weight.

Ingredients *(4 to 6 servings)*

2 sweet potatoes, peeled and cut into large pieces
½ tsp (3 ml) yellow curry paste
2 cups (500 ml) cooked brown rice
1 large egg, beaten, divided into 2 equal amounts
2 tbsp (30 ml) olive oil
2 shallots, chopped
1 tsp (5 ml) curry powder
½ tsp (2 ml) ground coriander
½ tsp (2 ml) ground cumin
1 clove of garlic, minced
8-oz (227-g) package of white mushrooms, chopped
salt and pepper to taste

Instructions

- Cook sweet potatoes in boiling water for about 12 minutes, until tender.
- Drain, then mash sweet potato, mixing in the curry paste.
- Let cool and set aside.
- Preheat oven to 350ºF (180ºC).
- Mix one half of the beaten egg with the rice.
- Spread out and flatten the rice mixture along the bottom and sides of a deep, buttered pie dish. Set aside.
- Heat the olive oil in a large pot. Sauté the shallots, spices, garlic and seasoning, without browning.
- Add mushrooms and cook for a few minutes until the liquid is absorbed.
- Let cool, then stir in the remaining half of the beaten egg.
- Combine the sweet potato and mushroom mixtures.
- Using a spoon, carefully transfer the pie filling to the dish.
- Cook in the oven for 25 minutes until the pie is firm. Serve warm.

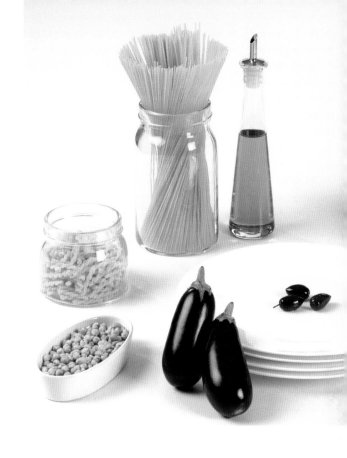

Main Courses

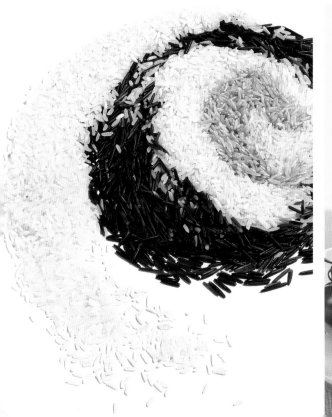

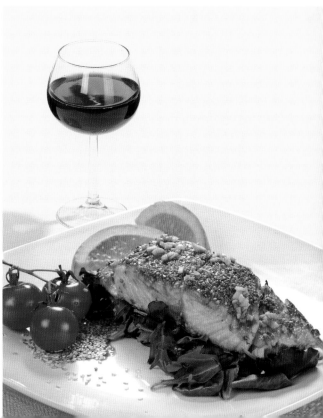

Main Course Masterpieces

Generally considered the centerpiece of any fine meal, the main course is more often than not a meat dish that is overly rich in fats and protein. Indeed, many people believe there is really no other way of preparing and presenting a substantial and satisfying meal.

Although meat dishes are not included in this book, we do not discourage meat. Animal protein and nutrients are unquestionably important for a healthy diet. Most health professionals, however, do not consider meat a healing food that is critically important to a well-balanced diet. Rather, it is one of several 'pillars' that sustain our body's good health. Furthermore, since most of us already eat adequate amounts of meat, we have chosen to exclude it as an ingredient from the recipes in this book. Our goal is to encourage people to eat more of the foods that contain important health-giving nutrients we are not getting enough of.

We hope that the following selection of recipes for main course dishes will counter the old notion that anything nutritious must fill the stomach. A main course can be satisfying and filling without being heavy and greasy. Recipes can be chosen to contain a greater variety of nutrients, vitamins and minerals; the main course does not have to be the traditional daily overloading of animal protein that so many people still believe, by force of habit, to be a 'proper' main course.

Main Course Recipes

(continued)

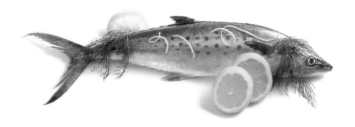

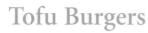

Tofu Burgers

Tofu is rich in calcium as well as in protein. These burgers are light and deliciously flavored with fennel seeds and tahini—a tasty, healthy change from regular ground-meat hamburgers.

Ingredients *(4 servings)*

½ lb (250 g) firm tofu
¼ cup (60 ml) tahini*
2 tbsp (30 ml) olive oil
1 onion, finely chopped
6 mushrooms, finely chopped
2 small carrots, unpeeled, grated
1 tsp (5 ml) fennel seeds, ground
⅓ cup (75 ml) unsalted sunflower seeds, finely crushed
¼ cup (60 ml) breadcrumbs
1 tbsp (15 ml) soy sauce or tamari
salt and pepper to taste

* Tahini is a purée made from sesame seeds, found in many specialty and health food shops.

Instructions

- Place tofu in a sieve or strainer to drain. Let sit for 30 minutes, then pat dry with a towel.
- Mix tofu to a paste or purée in a blender or food processor.
- Add tahini and mix to a smooth consistency.
- In a large saucepan, heat the oil and sauté the onion for a few minutes without browning. Add mushrooms and carrots and cook for 5 minutes or until carrots are tender.
- Add the vegetables to the tofu mixture in the blender. Add fennel, sunflower seeds, bread-crumbs and soy sauce.
- Season to taste, then process the mixture until ingredients are fully mixed and form into a ball.
- Divide the ball into 4 burger patties.
- Fry in a little oil or non-hydrogenated margarine for 5 to 8 minutes, turning only once, so that they are golden brown on the outside and warm inside.
- Serve each burger in a kaiser roll or between two slices of rye bread, garnished with slices of tomato and chèvre (goat cheese) that have been heated on the grill or under the broiler.

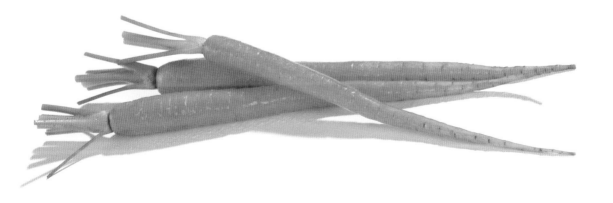

Millet Burgers

These delicious burgers have a nutty flavor and are a favorite with children. Millet is rich in silica, a mineral with beneficial effects on blood cholesterol and bone development.

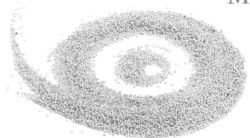

Ingredients *(4 servings)*

1 ½ cups (375 ml) cooked millet*
½ cup (125 ml) natural peanut butter
2 tbsp (30 ml) soy sauce or tamari
2 shallots, chopped
¼ tsp (1 ml) cumin or Maghrebian spice (see page 248)
4 kaiser rolls

* You can save time by cooking the millet the night before. Millet cooks like rice: two parts water to one part millet for 25 minutes or until liquid has been absorbed.

Instructions

- Mix all ingredients together and form into 4 burger patties.
- In a pan, heat a little oil or un-hydrogenated margarine over medium heat and fry patties for 2 minutes. Carefully turn them (they may be fragile), and continue to cook for 2 more minutes.
- Halve the kaiser rolls and place a patty in each one.
- Reheat in the oven or toaster oven, and serve with a crisp green salad.

Chick-Pea Burgers

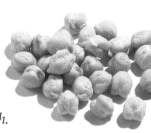

These meatless patties have a lovely seasoning and are a tasty way to include more legumes in your diet. They are a great source of dietary fiber, offering protection against cardiovascular disease, the world's number one cause of death.

Ingredients *(4 servings)*

2 cups (500 ml) canned chick-peas, rinsed and drained
2 shallots, finely minced
2 tbsp (30 ml) tahini*
¼ cup (60 ml) crushed vegetable crackers or bread-crumbs
¼ cup (60 ml) pecans, chopped
½ tsp (2 ml) Maghrebian spice (see page 248)
4 kaiser rolls

* Tahini is a purée made from sesame seeds, found in many specialty and health food shops.

Instructions

- In a food processor, mix the drained chick-peas to a paste.
- Add the remaining ingredients (except for the rolls) and mix again.
- Form the mixture into 4 burger patties and cook in a pan with a little olive oil or unhydrogenated margarine for 2 minutes on each side.
- Cut kaiser rolls in half and put a patty in each. Reheat in the oven or a toaster oven and serve with slices of tomato and lettuce.

Lentil Curry with Pistachio

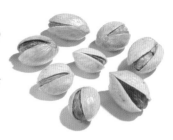

Perfumed with Indian spices, this dish is excellent as a light but nutritious meal, but it can also be served alongside grilled fish or meat. Since it provides a healthy amount of fiber, it makes for an effective protection against cardiovascular disease.

Ingredients *(4 servings)*

1 ½ cups (375 ml) green lentils, rinsed and drained

2 tbsp (30 ml) grapeseed oil (or sunflower or peanut oil)

2 onions, chopped

1 carrot, diced

1 zucchini, diced

1 cup (250 ml) sliced mushrooms, preferably shiitake

1 tsp (5 ml) fresh ginger, minced

1 tsp (5 ml) cumin

1 tsp (5 ml) turmeric

1 clove of garlic, minced

1 tsp (5 ml) salt

¼ tsp (1 ml) ground cloves

¼ tsp (1 ml) cinnamon

¼ tsp (1 ml) crushed chili peppers

1 ½ cups (375 ml) tomatoes (canned or fresh), chopped

⅓ cup (75 ml) green onion, chopped

¼ cup (60 ml) pistachios (shelled), coarsely chopped

¼ cup (60 ml) fresh coriander (cilantro), chopped

Instructions

- In a large pot, bring 5 cups (1.25 liters) of water to a boil, with the lentils. Reduce heat, cover and let simmer for 20 to 30 minutes or until lentils are tender.
- Drain and set aside.
- In another large pot, heat the grapeseed oil and sauté the onion, carrot, zucchini, mushrooms, ginger, garlic, salt, spices and chili flakes for 2 or 3 minutes.
- Add the tomatoes and cook over low heat for 20 minutes or until carrots are tender.
- Add the drained lentils and let simmer for 3 minutes. Mix in the green onion, pistachios and coriander. Serve hot.

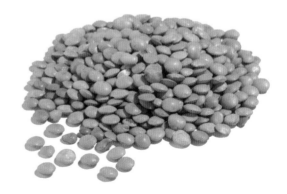

Barley Casserole au Gratin

This appetizing casserole is good for reducing the level of "bad" (LDL) cholesterol in the blood. It is a complete meal and another healthy substitute for a main course of meat. Children will enjoy this dish even more if almonds or walnuts are added.

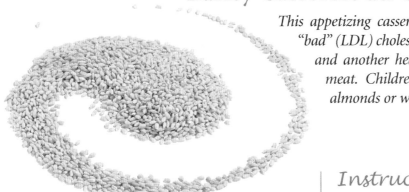

Ingredients *(4 servings)*

½ cup (125 ml) hulled whole barley
2 tbsp (30 ml) olive oil
2 shallots, finely minced
1 clove of garlic, minced
¾ cup (180 ml) sliced mushrooms
1 ½ cups (375 ml) tomatoes (canned or fresh), crushed
1 cup (250 ml) lentils, cooked
1 tsp (5 ml) mixed spices (coriander, cumin, chili pepper, fennel)
½ tsp (2 ml) mixture of dried oregano and basil
¼ cup (60 ml) fresh parsley, finely chopped
salt and pepper to taste
¾ cup (180 ml) grated Gruyere or strong cheddar cheese
¼ cup (60 ml) almonds or walnuts, chopped

Instructions

- Wash the barley, put in a large pot, cover with cold water and soak for 3 hours.
- Cook the barley in its soaking water over very low heat* for about 30 minutes.
- Meanwhile, prepare the sauce. In a large, oven-safe saucepan or casserole dish, sauté the shallot and garlic in the oil, then add mushrooms.
- Add tomatoes, lentils and spices and bring to a boil. Lower heat and let simmer, covered, for 20 minutes.
- Drain the barley and add to the other ingredients in the casserole dish.
- Add parsley, season to taste and mix well.
- Sprinkle the cheese and nuts over the casserole.
- Bake at 350ºF (180ºC) for about 30 minutes or until golden brown.

* Take care to lower the heat as soon as the barley is in the water; it will boil over easily.

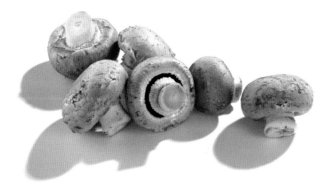

Kidney Bean and Lentil Casserole

This uniquely flavored dish—also known as Indian chili since it combines kidney beans with curry spices—is chock full of protein and dietary fiber. Along with being a fortifying protection against cardiovascular disease, it is, quite simply, delicious.

Ingredients *(4 servings)*

2 tbsp (30 ml) olive oil
1 onion, finely chopped
1 zucchini, diced
1 clove of garlic, minced
19-oz (540-ml) can of kidney beans
19-oz (540-ml) can of lentils
1 egg
1 carrot (unpeeled), grated
¾ cup (180 ml) cheddar cheese
½ cup (125 ml) breadcrumbs
2 tbsp (30 ml) salsa
1 tsp (5ml) of each of the following: cumin, coriander, ground fennel, chili
salt and pepper to taste

Instructions

- Preheat oven to 350ºF (180ºC).
- Butter or oil a casserole dish or cake pan large enough to hold all the ingredients.
- In a large pot, sauté the onion and zucchini in the oil for about 5 minutes without browning.
- Add garlic, stir and set aside.
- Rinse the kidney beans and lentils, drain well and place in a large mixing bowl.
- Add onion-zucchini mixture to the beans, then add all remaining ingredients except for ¼ cup (60 ml) of the cheese. Mix carefully, season to taste, then pour into the greased casserole dish, flattening the surface. Sprinkle with the remaining cheese.
- Cook for 45 minutes.

Variation

Consider serving this dish as an appetizer instead of fat-rich cold cuts or pâté de fois gras. For this, mix the beans and lentils in a food processor before cooking, and refrigerate the casserole to be served chilled.

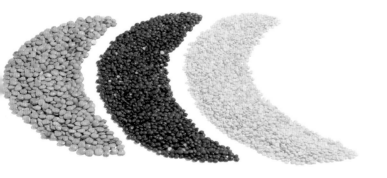

Vegetable Chick-Pea Casserole au Gratin

This tasty dish of vegetables and legumes is enhanced with oats, walnuts and cheese. It is a marvelous, hearty winter food that supplies an abundance of fiber and vitamins.

Ingredients *(4 servings)*

1 leek, chopped
2 carrots (unpeeled), diced
3 turnips, diced
1 sweet potato, diced
2 stalks of celery, diced
3 tbsp (45 ml) olive oil
1 tsp (5ml) ground coriander
1 tsp (5 ml) herbs Provençal (marjoram, thyme, basil, rosemary, savory)
1 clove of garlic, minced
1 lb (454 g) tomatoes, seeded, crushed
1 vegetable stock cube
¼ cup (60 ml) unsweetened evaporated milk
19-oz (540-ml) can of chick-peas
salt and pepper to taste

Topping

¼ cup (60 ml) rolled oats
¼ cup (60 ml) vegetable crackers, finely crushed
¼ cup (60 ml) walnuts
½ cup (125 ml) grated cheese
2 tbsp (30 ml) clarified butter
(see page 152)

Instructions

- Preheat oven to 375ºF (190ºC).
- In an oven-safe casserole dish or baking dish, sauté the leek, carrot, turnip, sweet potato and celery in olive oil for 5 minutes on the stovetop.
- Add the coriander, herbs, garlic, crumbled stock cube and tomatoes, and bring to a boil.
- Reduce heat and let simmer for 10 minutes.
- Add evaporated milk and chick-peas and season to taste. Simmer for 10 minutes more.
- Prepare the topping by mixing the cracker crumbs, nuts, rolled oats, grated cheese and butter.
- Spread the topping over the surface of the vegetable mixture.
- Cook in the oven for 15 minutes.

Eggplant Chili

This easy-to-make, flavorful chili dish marvelously combines vegetables possessing antioxidant properties with protein-rich kidney beans—a health-giving partnership that is topped off with chili powder, an effective remedy for relieving arthritis.

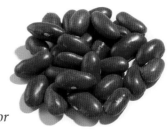

Ingredients *(4 servings)*

2 tbsp (30 ml) olive oil
1 onion, minced
1 clove of garlic, minced
1 small sweet red pepper, diced
2 medium zucchinis, cubed
1 small eggplant, cubed
19-oz (540-ml) can of kidney beans, rinsed and drained
2 tbsp (30 ml) chili powder, or to taste
1 cup (250 ml) or more, vegetable juice* or Homemade Vegetable Broth (see page 166)
salt and pepper to taste

* Canned vegetable cocktail also makes an excellent liquid for this chili recipe.

Instructions

- In a large pot, sauté the onion and garlic in the oil for 1 or 2 minutes to tenderize without browning.
- Add red pepper, zucchini and eggplant. Cook for another 2 minutes, stirring constantly.
- Add beans, chili powder and enough vegetable juice or broth to cover the mixture.
- Bring to a boil, then reduce heat and let simmer, covered, for 30 minutes.
- Remove lid, correct seasoning, add more pepper and chili powder if you prefer a spicier chili; cook for another 15 minutes. Cook uncovered if the sauce has not thickened sufficiently.

Tofu Chili

This delicious, meatless chili is rich in protein, calcium and fiber, and protects the body against cardiovascular disease.

Ingredients *(4 servings)*

1 tbsp (15 ml) olive oil
1 onion, chopped
1 red or orange sweet pepper, diced
1 zucchini, diced
1 clove of garlic, minced
1 cup (250 ml) tomato sauce, canned or, even better, homemade (see page 226)
1 cup (250 ml) Homemade Vegetable Broth (see page 166)
19-oz (540-ml) can of kidney beans, rinsed and drained
2 tbsp (30 ml) chili powder, or to taste
12-oz (350-g) package of firm tofu, broken up with a fork
salt and pepper to taste

Instructions

- In a large pot, heat the oil and sauté the onion, sweet pepper, and zucchini without browning.
- Add garlic, tomato sauce, vegetable broth, kidney beans, chili powder and seasoning. Cook for 40 minutes.
- Add the tofu and continue to heat for another few minutes before serving.

Salmon Steaks with Green Pepper*
(microwave recipe)

This lightning-fast way of cooking fish ensures that the flesh remains tender, moist and delicate. It works as well for trout and salmon-trout as for salmon, all of which are cold-water fish rich in beneficial omega-3 fatty acids.

Ingredients *(4 servings)*

4 salmon steaks
2 tbsp (30 ml) butter
2 tbsp (30 ml) lemon juice
zest of ½ lemon
2 tbsp (30 ml) green peppercorns (preserved in brine)
salt and pepper to taste

Instructions

- Using a microwave-safe dish large enough to hold the 4 salmon steaks, melt the butter in the microwave for 1 minute.
- Add lemon juice, zest and green pepper, and mix well. Add the salmon steaks, turning them over once, ensuring that they are well coated in the mixture.
- Place dish in microwave and cook salmon at 70 percent for 3 minutes. Turn steaks over and cook for another 2 minutes.
- Check salmon and cook slightly longer if necessary. Cooking time will vary according to the thickness of the salmon and the type of microwave oven. Let sit for 3 minutes before serving.

* Green peppercorns are from the same plant that produces black pepper; not green bell or sweet peppers.

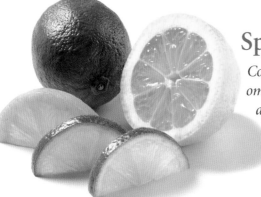

Spicy Fish Fillets

Cold-water 'fatty' fish, such as salmon or mackerel, contain omega-3 fatty acids that, among other benefits, slow the effects of aging. This simple and delicious preparation of fish fillets works well with most white fish.

Ingredients *(4 servings)*

1 lb (500 g) fresh white fish fillets of your choice
2 eggs, beaten
1 tsp (5 ml) mixture of crushed chili, ground coriander, cumin powder, ground fennel and cardamom
½ cup (125 ml) breadcrumbs
2 tbsp (30 ml) clarified butter (see page 152), non-hydrogenated margarine or grapeseed oil
juice and zest of ½ lemon
salt and pepper to taste

Préparation

- Place fish fillets on a large sheet of wax paper.
- Put the beaten eggs in a bowl large enough to bread the fillets.
- Mix the breadcrumbs, lemon zest and spices in another large bowl.
- Heat the butter, margarine or oil in a large pan.
- Dip one fillet into the beaten egg to coat well, then into the breadcrumb mixture. Repeat with all four fillets.
- Fry fillets in the pan, season to taste, sprinkle with lemon juice and serve hot.

Salmon Fillets with Sesame

Topped with an orange and ginger sauce, these salmon fillets are prepared in a snap. Atlantic salmon, in particular, is rich in omega-3, a compound that regulates blood pressure and preserves the arteries.

Ingredients *(4 servings)*

4 salmon fillets (about ¼ lb, or 125 g, each)
1 tbsp (15 ml) liquid honey
1 tbsp (15 ml) soy sauce or tamari
1 tbsp (15 ml) Dijon mustard
1 tbsp (15 ml) grapeseed oil (or other light oil)
2 tbsp (30 ml) sesame seeds
mixed lettuce leaves to cover 4 plates, washed and spun

Vinaigrette

1 clove of garlic, minced
1 tsp (5 ml) fresh ginger, minced
3 tbsp (45 ml) orange juice
2 tsp (10 ml) soy sauce or tamari
2 tsp (10 ml) balsamic vinegar
2 tsp (10 ml) sesame oil
a few drops of chili sauce

Instructions

- Preheat oven to 425°F (220°C).
- Pat the fillets dry with a paper towel and set aside.
- Mix together the honey, soy sauce, mustard and oil in a bowl. One at a time, dip the fillets into this mixture to coat them well. Sprinkle with sesame seeds.
- In a large non-stick frying pan, lightly brown the fish fillets over medium-high heat for 1 minute on each side.
- Arrange fillets in a baking dish, cook in the oven for 7 to 8 minutes more.
- Meanwhile, prepare the vinaigrette. Beat together the garlic, ginger, orange juice, soy sauce, vinegar, sesame oil and chili sauce.
- Arrange lettuce leaves on the 4 serving plates. As soon as the fish is cooked, place one fillet on each bed of lettuce, sprinkle with vinaigrette and serve.

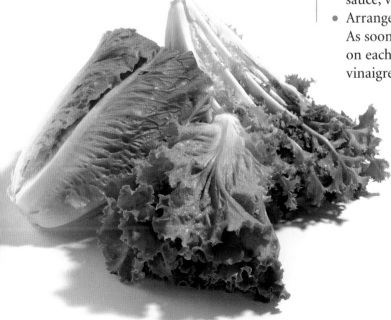

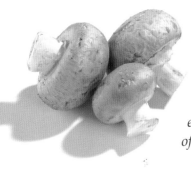

Spinach and Mushroom Lasagna

This meatless lasagna is not only delicious and nutritious, it also offers excellent protection against "bad" (LDL) cholesterol as well as various kinds of infection.

Ingredients *(4 servings)*

6 to 9 lasagna noodles

Sauce

¼ cup (60 ml) clarified butter (see page 152)
¼ cup (60 ml) flour
2 cups (500 ml) milk (2%)
½ onion, left whole
salt and pepper to taste

Filling

2 tbsp (30 ml) olive oil
1 shallot, minced
8-oz (227-g) package of mushrooms, chopped
1 clove of garlic, minced
10-oz (284-g) package of spinach, washed and dried, larger stems removed, chopped
¼ cup (60 ml) hazelnuts, coarsely chopped
1 pinch of nutmeg
¾ cup (180 ml) grated Gruyere cheese
salt and pepper to taste

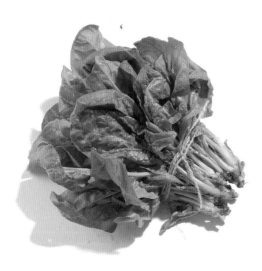

Instructions

- Preheat oven to 375ºF (190ºC).
- Cook lasagna noodles in boiling water until *al dente*, following instructions on package. Drain and let cool. Prepare the white sauce while the noodles are cooking and cooling.
- In a small pot, heat the butter until melted, then stir in the flour. Add the half onion (for flavor) and milk, and cook over medium heat until sauce thickens.
- Remove and discard the onion. Season sauce to taste and let cool.
- To prepare the filling, sauté the shallot in the olive oil without browning.
- Add mushrooms and garlic. Cook until the moisture from the mushrooms has evaporated.
- Add spinach, hazelnuts and nutmeg, and cook until the spinach has softened in the steam. Taste and adjust seasoning.
- Arrange a third of the lasagna noodles in a layer on the bottom of a buttered or oiled 7 in. by 12 in. (18 cm by 30 cm) baking pan.
- Spread half of the spinach mixture over the noodles. Add a layer of half the white sauce.
- Add a second layer of lasagna noodles, then a layer of the remaining spinach mixture.
- Finish with a third layer of lasagna noodles and the remaining white sauce. Top with the grated cheese.
- Cook in the oven for 35 minutes or until the surface just begins to brown.

Linguine with Almond

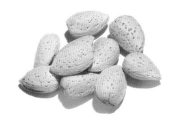

The orange, ginger and grilled almonds in this dish lend their flavors to the tofu—a food which has no flavor at all but is versatile in cooking. It also contains a full array of protein, calcium and other nutrients that more than compensate for its lack of taste.

Ingredients *(4 servings)*

1 tbsp (15 ml) olive oil
2 cloves of garlic, minced
1 leek, chopped
1 cup (250 ml) mushrooms, chopped
½ sweet red pepper, diced
1 carrot, grated
½ cup (125 ml) Homemade Vegetable or Chicken Broth (see pages 165 and 166)
2 tbsp (30 ml) tamari sauce, or soy sauce if unavailable
1 tsp (5 ml) grated fresh ginger
zest of 1 orange
1 cup (250 ml) tofu, broken or chopped into small pieces
½ cup (125 ml) flaked almonds, grilled (in the oven at 350ºF, or 180ºC, for 7 to 9 minutes)
¾ lb (375 g) linguine pasta, cooked (in salt water) *al dente*
salt and pepper to taste

Instructions

- In a large pot, heat the oil and sauté the leek without browning.
- Add garlic, mushrooms, sweet pepper, carrot, broth, tamari sauce and ginger. Mix well to coat the vegetables.
- Cover and bring to a boil. Reduce heat and simmer for 5 minutes or until the mushrooms are tender.
- Add tofu and orange zest and stir gently.
- Cover and simmer for 5 more minutes.
- Sprinkle with the flaked almonds.
- If the sauce is too thin, thicken with a little cornstarch dissolved in a spoonful or two of water.
- Serve over the linguine.

Variation

For a Mediterranean flavor, replace the carrot, orange zest and ginger with sun-dried tomatoes, chopped fresh basil and coarsely chopped, pitted black olives.

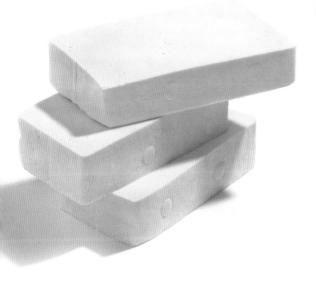

Pasta Puttanesca

This famous pasta dish is a tasty way to benefit from the antiviral properties of garlic.

Ingredients *(4 servings)*

1 lb (454 g) short pasta (such as fusilli or penne), cooked
¼ cup (60 ml) olive oil
15 to 20 black olives, pitted and chopped
6 anchovy fillets, finely chopped, mixed with
1 tbsp (15 ml) butter
2 cloves of garlic, minced
1 tbsp (15 ml) capers, rinsed, drained and chopped
1 ½ cups (375 ml) fresh tomatoes, peeled, seeded and crushed (or canned crushed tomatoes)
¼ cup (60 ml) fresh parsley, chopped
freshly ground black pepper

Instructions

- Heat the oil on medium and sauté the olives, anchovies, garlic and capers for 2 minutes.
- Add the tomatoes and bring to a boil. Lower the heat and simmer for 20 minutes covered.
- Mix the sauce with the cooked pasta, sprinkle with the parsley, season to taste and serve hot.

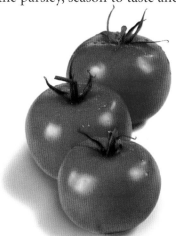

Pizza with Sockeye Salmon and Fresh Vegetables

These small pizzas are quick to prepare and can also be served as an appetizer. They are much healthier than any frozen pizza and do not take much longer to prepare. The salmon is a great source of omega-3 fatty acids.

Ingredients *(4 servings)*

4 corn- or wheat-flour tortillas, ready to eat
2 fresh tomatoes, seeded, crushed and drained (or substitute ¼ cup, or 60 ml, of pizza sauce)
7 ½-oz (213-g) can of sockeye salmon, drained and flaked
12 to 16 mushrooms, finely sliced
12 to 16 black olives, pitted and chopped
1 cup (250 ml) grated Gruyere cheese

Instructions

- Preheat oven to 450ºF (230ºC).
- Place the tortillas on a baking sheet or on small individual pizza pans.
- Garnish each with crushed tomatoes or pizza sauce, flaked salmon, mushroom slices and chopped olives.
- Cover with grated cheese.
- Cook in the oven for 6 to 7 minutes until the cheese just begins to brown.

Quiche with Millet, Tofu and Lentils

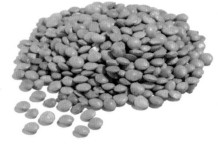

This delicious cheese-filled quiche is rich in protein, fiber and calcium: a tasty dish that protects against cardiovascular illnesses.

Ingredients *(4 to 6 servings)*

Crust

¾ cup (180 ml) cooked millet
¾ cup (180 ml) grated cheese
1 small egg, beaten

Filling

2 tbsp (30 ml) olive oil
1 shallot, chopped
1 clove of garlic, minced
½ sweet red pepper, diced
½ sweet orange pepper, diced
1 cup (250 ml) lentils, cooked
1 zucchini, cubed
1 tsp (5 ml) curry powder
½ tsp (2 ml) ground fennel seeds
½ tsp (2 ml) ground coriander
½ tsp (2 ml) turmeric
¼ cup (60 ml) table cream (15%)
4 oz (225 g) block of plain tofu, diced
1 egg, lightly beaten

Topping

¾ cup (180 ml) cooked millet
¾ cup (180 ml) grated cheese
¼ cup (60 ml) pine nuts

Instructions

- Grease a quiche dish or deep pie dish with butter and line with the crust mixture made from the cooked millet, grated cheese and egg. Press down gently to cover the base of the dish.
- In a saucepan, sauté the shallot, garlic and sweet peppers in the oil for a few minutes without browning.
- Add lentils, zucchini and spices and let cook for 15 minutes, adding a little water or broth as necessary to keep the mixture moist.
- Remove from heat, let cool, then add the diced tofu, cream and beaten egg.
- Stir filling to mix well. Gently pour into the quiche or pie dish.
- Mix together the topping ingredients and spread evenly over the quiche.
- Bake at 350ºF (180ºC) for 30 minutes.

Cooking Tip

Cook the millet the night before, and cook a little extra so as to have some ready at hand to add to soups and stews.

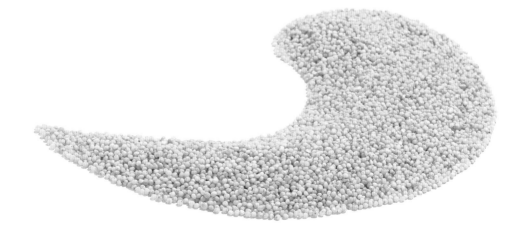

Vegetable Feta Cheese Quiche
with Pecan Crust

The combination of mushroom, spinach and zucchini with a mixture of egg, milk and cheese makes for a healthy meal full of calcium and fortifying, beneficial ingredients.

Ingredients *(4 to 6 servings)*

2 tbsp (30 ml) non-hydrogenated margarine
¾ cup (180 ml) mixture of chopped pecans and crushed vegetable crackers
1 tbsp (15 ml) olive oil
1 leek (white part only), chopped
1 cup (250 ml) mushrooms, sliced
1 cup (250 ml) zucchini, chopped
3 cups (750 ml) fresh spinach, chopped
2 eggs
1 cup (250 ml) unsweetened evaporated milk
⅔ cup (150 ml) feta cheese, crumbled
2 tbsp (30 ml) fresh basil, chopped (or
1 tsp / 5 ml dried)
dash of hot sauce, to taste

Variation

The feta cheese can be replaced by Gruyere cheese, if desired. In this case, the cooking time should be shortened by 10 minutes and the egg mixture should be salted slightly since Gruyere contains much less salt than feta cheese.

Préparation

- Preheat oven to 350°F (180°C).
- Grease a microwave-safe quiche dish or 10-in (25-cm) pie plate with a little margarine. Mix the rest of the margarine with the pecans and cracker crumbs. Line the quiche dish with this mixture.
- Cook crust for 2 minutes in the microwave* at medium-high (70%) intensity.
- In a non-stick saucepan, heat the olive oil and sauté the leek, mushroom and zucchini for about 7 minutes or until vegetables are tender and the liquid has evaporated.
- Add the spinach and cook for 2 more minutes.
- Beat the eggs in a large bowl, then mix in the milk. Continue to stir while adding the feta cheese, basil and a dash of hot sauce.
- Transfer the vegetable mixture to the quiche dish, then top with the egg-cheese mixture.
- Bake for 40 to 50 minutes or until the surface is golden brown.

* Or in a conventional oven for 15 minutes at 350°F (180°C).

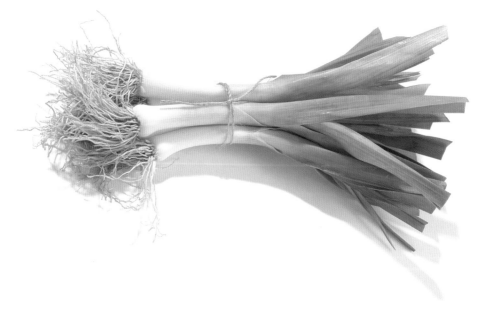

Chinese Cabbage Rolls

This hearty dish brings together several healing foods that help the body protect itself against cardiovascular disease.

Ingredients *(4 servings)*

12 large leaves of Chinese cabbage
1 ½ cups (375 ml) cooked wild rice or quinoa
⅔ cup (150 ml) pecans, coarsely chopped
1 tomato (seeds removed), diced
2 small sweet red peppers, grilled (see page 95), diced
1 tsp (5 ml) Harissa Chili Sauce (see page 223)
salt and pepper to taste

Mushroom Sauce

1 tbsp (15 ml) olive oil
1 shallot, chopped
1 clove of garlic, minced
8-oz (227-g) package of white mushrooms
3 tbsp (45 ml) butter
3 tbsp (45 ml) flour
1 ½ cups (375 ml) Homemade Chicken Broth (see page 165)
1 tbsp (15 ml) Worcestershire sauce
1 tsp (2 ml) black pepper

Instructions

- Preheat oven to 350ºF (180ºC).
- In a large pot, heat enough water to cook the cabbage leaves whole.
- Meanwhile, prepare the filling by mixing together the rice or quinoa, pecans, tomato, sweet pepper and chili sauce.
- Add the cabbage leaves to the boiling water, cooking each for 1 minute, then dropping them into ice water. Drain in a strainer.
- Pat dry the cabbage leaves, remove any excess length of stem, then spoon about 3 to 4 tbsp (45 to 60 ml) of filling onto the widest part of each leaf.
- Carefully roll up each leaf to form a cabbage roll and secure with a toothpick, if necessary. Repeat with all 12 cabbage leaves. Arrange rolls in a greased baking dish and bake for 15 minutes.
- Meanwhile, prepare mushroom sauce by heating the oil. Sauté the shallot, add the garlic and mushroom and cook until reduced by half. Remove from the saucepan and set aside. Melt the butter and mix in the flour. Add the broth, Worcestershire sauce and pepper. Add mushroom mixture and stir over medium heat until sauce thickens.
- Once cabbage rolls have heated, pour the mushroom sauce over and serve. Goes superbly with Mashed Potatoes with Carrot and Rutabaga (see page 184).

Spaghetti with Meatless Bolognaise Sauce

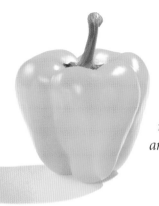

This pasta sauce seems just like a meat sauce; in fact many of your dinner guests might not even notice that it contains no meat. Yet, since it's much lower in calories, this is a healthier substitute that also supplies an appreciable amount of protein, dietary fiber and vitamins.

Ingredients *(4 to 6 servings)*

1 large onion, finely chopped
2 tbsp (30 ml) olive oil
8-oz (225-g) block of regular tofu, finely chopped*
1 sweet red or orange pepper, diced
1 carrot, scrubbed and diced
1 zucchini, washed (unpeeled), cut into pieces
8-oz (225-g) package white mushrooms, chopped
2 cloves of garlic, minced
28-oz (796 ml) can of crushed tomatoes
5 ½-oz (156-ml) can tomato paste
1 tsp (5 ml) dried basil
1 tsp (5 ml) dried oregano
2 tsp (10 ml) chili powder
1 tsp (5 ml) chili flakes
1 cup (250 ml) vegetable juice
2 bay leaves
salt and pepper to taste

Instructions

- In a large pot, heat the olive oil and sauté the onion without browning.
- Add the tofu and cook for a few minutes. Mince any larger pieces of tofu with the spatula.
- Add the other vegetables, tomatoes, tomato paste, herbs, spices and vegetable juice.
- Adjust seasoning with salt and pepper. Let sauce simmer, covered, for 1 hour.
- Serve over spaghetti or other pasta, on rice or over a dish of cooked vegetables.

*   The tofu should be very finely minced to pass for meat in this sauce, and to absorb all of the flavors.

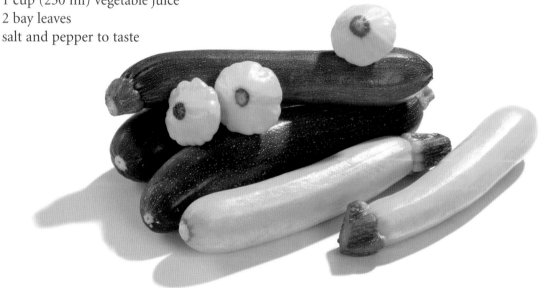

Spaghetti with Eggplant and Shiitake Mushrooms

This delicious spaghetti sauce brings together a variety of vegetables from our list of healing foods. Together, they contribute rich flavors and aromas that will make you completely forget that the dish contains no meat.

Ingredients *(4 to 6 servings)*

2 tbsp (30 ml) olive oil
1 onion, minced
1 sweet red or orange pepper, diced
2 carrots, scrubbed and diced
1 zucchini, washed (unpeeled), diced
1 celery stalk, diced
1 parsnip, scrubbed and diced
1 medium eggplant, washed (unpeeled), diced
8 fresh shiitake mushrooms, chopped
2 cloves of garlic, minced
2 28-oz (796-ml) cans of crushed tomatoes
¼ cup (60 ml) tomato paste
1 tsp (5 ml) dried basil
1 tsp (5 ml) dried oregano
1 tsp (5 ml) herbs Provençal (marjoram, thyme, basil, rosemary, savory)
1 tsp (5 ml) chili flakes
2 bay leaves
salt and pepper to taste
cooked spaghetti

Instructions

- In a large pot, sauté the onion in the oil for a few minutes without browning, then add sweet peppers, carrot, zucchini and celery.
- Cook for another few minutes, stirring continuously.
- Add the parsnip, eggplant and all remaining sauce ingredients and bring to a boil.
- Lower the heat and let simmer over low heat for 1 hour.
- Serve sauce over spaghetti, dusted with freshly grated parmesan cheese.

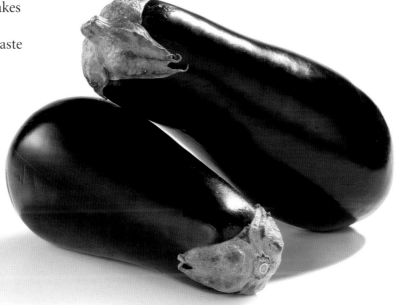

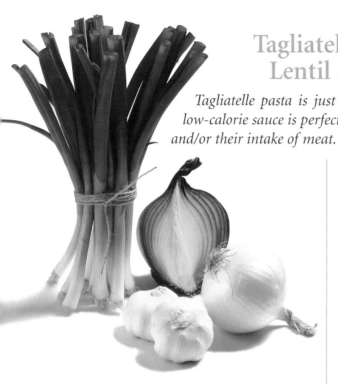

Tagliatelle with Lentil Sauce

Tagliatelle pasta is just slightly narrower than fettucine. This delicious, low-calorie sauce is perfect for people trying to reduce their cholesterol levels and/or their intake of meat.

Instructions

- In a large pot, heat olive oil and sauté the onion without browning.
- Add carrots and celery and cook for 3 minutes.
- Add garlic, lentils and chicken broth and bring to a boil.
- Lower the heat and let simmer, covered, for 1 hour.
- Add the remaining ingredients (except pasta) and bring to a boil. Lower the heat and simmer for another 15 minutes.
- Serve over tagliatelle or other long pasta.

Ingredients *(6 servings)*

2 tbsp (30 ml) olive oil
2 onions, minced
2 small carrots, diced
2 stalks of celery, diced
2 cloves of garlic, minced
1 cup (250 ml) dry lentils, rinsed and drained
2 cups (500 ml) Homemade Chicken Broth (see page 165)
½ cup (125 ml) red wine
3 tbsp (45 ml) tomato paste
¾ cup (180 ml) tomato sauce (see page 226)
4 oz (120 g) mushrooms, chopped
1 tsp (5 ml) dried oregano
1 tsp (5 ml) dried basil
cooked tagliatelle pasta

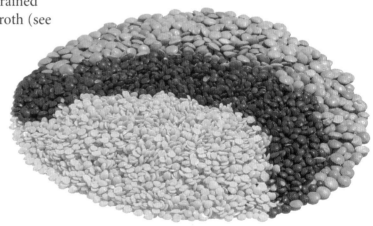

Barley Vege-Paté

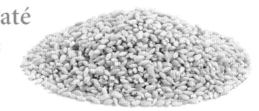

People who are recovering from illness or suffering from anemia will appreciate this hearty, highly digestible dish that is a fortifying restorative.

Ingredients

⅔ cup (150 ml) hulled whole barley
¼ cup (60 ml) wheat germ
¼ cup (60 ml) walnuts, chopped
⅓ cup (75 ml) unsalted sunflower seeds
1 small carrot, grated
1 small zucchini (unpeeled), grated
1 ½ cups (375 ml) Gruyere cheese, grated
1 tsp (5 ml) salt
freshly ground black pepper to taste
1 egg, lightly beaten
2 tbsp (30 ml) chopped fresh parsley

Instructions

- Cook the barley in 1 ¾ cups (430 ml) water for about 1 hour.
- Drain well, as necessary. If you prefer, uncooked barley can be soaked in cold water for a few hours, then cooked in its soaking water for 30 minutes.
- Once the barley is cooked, leave to cool.
- Preheat oven to 350ºF (180ºC).
- Mix the barley with all of the other ingredients in a large mixing bowl.
- Pour mixture into a 9-inch (23-cm) greased bread pan, pressing down gently.
- Bake in the oven for 40 minutes.
- Let cool for 10 minutes.
- Carefully remove from bread pan and slice. Serve topped with Fresh Tomato Sauce (see page 226).

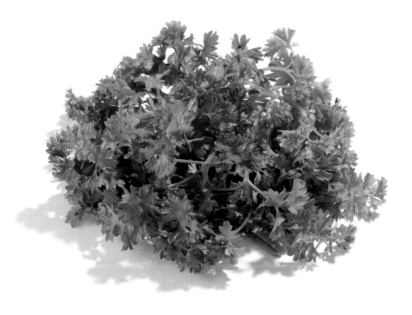

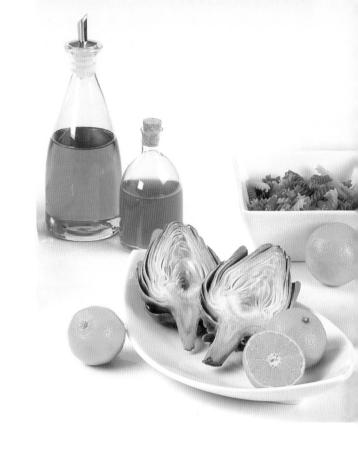

Mixed Salads

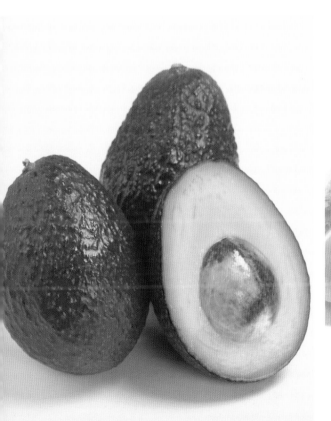

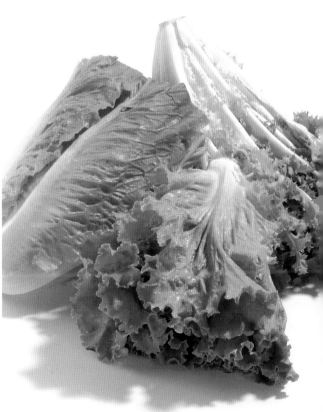

Mixed Salads:
Medical Wonders

A mixed salad, prepared with a full array of fresh ingredients, can be a complete meal unto itself. Salads have the advantage of combining low-calorie foods that are extremely beneficial to the body, helping it to fight off infections and protect against diseases. The composition of your salads can be easily adjusted according to the vegetables (and fruit) that are best for you at any given time. Have a look at the foods in Part One of this book to learn about some of the best combinations of salad ingredients offering health-boosting properties. Inspire yourself with the selection of recipes in this section, then start mixing and matching your own salads to best suit your particular health needs.

Salad Recipes

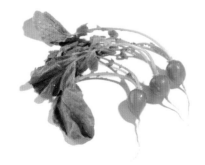

Salade Niçoise

This satisfying salad can be a meal in itself. Leave out the tuna and it is an appetizer that still retains many of its health-giving, preventive properties.

Ingredients *(4 servings)*

3 cups (750 ml) mixed salad greens, washed and dried

1 cup (250 ml) green beans, cooked *al dente*, cut in half

2 ripe tomatoes, seeded and crushed

12 black olives, pitted and chopped

1 small can of flaked tuna, drained

Vinaigrette

¼ cup (60 ml) olive oil

2 tbsp (30 ml) lemon juice

1 tbsp (15 ml) balsamic vinegar

1 small clove of garlic, minced

fresh basil, finely chopped

salt and pepper to taste

Instructions

- Combine salad greens, beans, tomatoes, olives and flaked tuna in a large bowl. Mix well.
- In a small bowl, whisk together the ingredients for the vinaigrette.
- Add the vinaigrette to the salad in a thin stream while mixing.
- Taste and adjust seasoning as necessary. Mix again and serve.

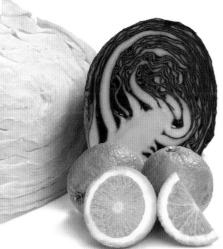

Cabbage Salad with Clementine, Spinach and Sesame

This salad is delicious at any time of the year. It is a fortifying tonic that combats fatigue and hypertension.

Ingredients *(4 servings)*

1 small whole cabbage, cut into 1-inch (2-cm) strips

4 clementines, peeled and cut into thin slices

15 to 20 spinach leaves, washed and dried

¼ cup (60 ml) grapeseed or sunflower oil

¼ cup (60 ml) walnut or peanut oil

2 tbsp (30 ml) lemon juice

zest of 1 lemon

a handful of sesame seeds, toasted

salt and pepper to taste

Instructions

- Combine the cabbage, slices of clementine and spinach leaves in a large bowl.
- Mix together the oils, lemon juice and zest in a smaller bowl. Add this vinaigrette to the salad in a thin stream while mixing.
- Refrigerate* for at least 30 minutes.
- Just before serving, add sesame seeds, season to taste and mix again.

* Cabbage becomes more digestible if refrigerated for at least half an hour (blended with the vinaigrette).

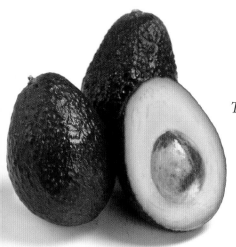

Artichoke Apple Avocado Salad

This elegant and nourishing salad brings together fruits and vegetables that are full of vitamins and minerals. The three flavors blend harmoniously in this satisfying, highly digestible salad appetizer.

Ingredients *(2 servings)*

¼ cup (60 ml) grapeseed or sunflower oil
3 tbsp (45 ml) lemon juice
zest of ½ lemon
1 clove of garlic, minced
2 tbsp (30 ml) fresh coriander (cilantro), finely chopped
salt and pepper to taste
1 cup (250 ml) sliced cabbage, cut into 1-inch (2-cm) strips
4 preserved artichoke hearts, cut in four
1 fully ripe avocado, cut into bite-size pieces
2 Empire apples, cubed

Instructions

- Prepare the vinaigrette by combining the oil, half the lemon juice, zest, garlic, coriander and seasoning.
- In a large salad bowl, pour vinaigrette over the cabbage, mix and refrigerate* for at least 30 minutes.
- Just before serving, add the artichoke hearts, avocado and apples, sprinkled with the remaining lemon juice.
- Mix again and serve.

* Cabbage becomes more digestible if refrigerated for at least half an hour (blended with the vinaigrette).

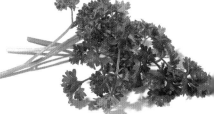

Couscous and Parsley Salad (Taboulé)

This Lebanese appetizer is a delicious way to include more parsley in your diet—an underappreciated herb rich in vitamins and minerals that also combats anemia.

Ingredients *(2 to 4 servings)*

2 well-packed cups (500 ml) minced fresh parsley (including stems)
1 cup (250 ml) couscous or quinoa, cooked according to package instructions*
2 small shallots, finely minced
2 medium tomatoes, seeded, crushed
4 to 6 tbsp (60 to 90 ml) olive oil
2 tbsp (30 ml) lemon juice
2 or 3 fresh mint leaves, finely minced

Instructions

- In a salad bowl, mix together all ingredients and let sit for 1 hour to allow full flavors to develop.

* Couscous (or wheat semolina) is usually cooked as follows: boil one part water with one part couscous. At the point of boiling, remove from heat. Let sit for 3 minutes, then add 1 tbsp (15 ml) olive oil and gently separate grains using a fork, reheating over low heat for about 2 minutes.

Fennel Salad with Orange

The aromas of aniseed, orange and coriander blend well in this salad, making it a refreshing appetizer served before a main course of meat.

Ingredients *(4 servings)*

2 cups (500 ml) salad greens, washed and dried
1 whole fennel bulb, cut into strips julienne-style
1 orange (zest and juice)
2 oranges (or 4 clementines), peeled, thinly sliced
1 small sweet onion, chopped (or 2 shallots, finely minced)
2 tbsp (30 ml) chopped fresh coriander (cilantro)
1 tbsp (15 ml) sesame seeds

Vinaigrette

2 tbsp (30 ml) grapeseed or sunflower oil
2 tbsp (30 ml) walnut or peanut oil
1 tbsp (15 ml) balsamic vinegar
salt and pepper to taste

Instructions

- Put fennel strips in a bowl and drizzle with the orange juice and zest. Add the orange slices and chopped onion. Mix gently and refrigerate for 1 hour.
- Prepare the vinaigrette by beating together ingredients with a whisk in a small bowl. Let sit.
- Put the salad greens in a bowl and add the refrigerated fennel-orange mixture. Mix well.
- Pour vinaigrette over the salad and mix again. Garnish with the fresh coriander and sesame seeds. Serve.

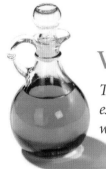

Vegetable Pasta Salad with Feta

This light meal, which can be made with leftover pasta, is composed of two excellent combinations of healing foods: tomatoes with spinach, and cheese with apple cider vinegar.

Ingredients *(4 servings)*

3 cups (750 ml) cooked short pasta (e.g. fusilli, macaroni, conchiglie, etc.), preferably vegetable or 'rainbow' pasta
2 tomatoes, seeded and crushed
¼ cup (60 ml) cooked spinach, chopped
¼ cup (60 ml) feta cheese,* crumbled
¼ cup (60 ml) black olives, pitted and chopped

* Be careful about the quantity of salt you add since the feta cheese and olives both contain considerable amounts of salt. If desired, replace the feta with a lower-calorie, less salty cheese such as chèvre (goat cheese) or cottage cheese.

Vinaigrette

¼ cup (60 ml) olive oil
2 tbsp (30 ml) apple cider vinegar
2 tbsp (30 ml) chopped fresh basil
salt* and pepper to taste

Instructions

- Prepare the vinaigrette by whisking together ingredients in a small bowl. Adjust seasoning.
- Combine all of the ingredients in a large bowl and blend well. Add the vinaigrette in a thin stream and mix again. Serve.

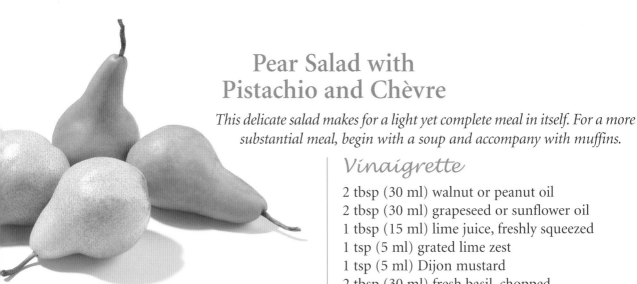

Pear Salad with Pistachio and Chèvre

This delicate salad makes for a light yet complete meal in itself. For a more substantial meal, begin with a soup and accompany with muffins.

Ingredients *(2 to 4 servings)*

2 cups (500 ml) mixed salad greens, washed and dried
2 fully ripe pears, peeled, cubed and sprinkled with lime juice
¼ cup (60 ml) pistachios, shelled, coarsely chopped
¼ cup (60 ml) chèvre (goat) cheese, diced

Variation

Replace the mixed salad greens with sliced cabbage and the chèvre cheese with feta.

Vinaigrette

2 tbsp (30 ml) walnut or peanut oil
2 tbsp (30 ml) grapeseed or sunflower oil
1 tbsp (15 ml) lime juice, freshly squeezed
1 tsp (5 ml) grated lime zest
1 tsp (5 ml) Dijon mustard
2 tbsp (30 ml) fresh basil, chopped
salt and pepper to taste

Instructions

- Put the mixed salad greens in a large salad bowl.
- Add the cubed pear, pistachio and chèvre cheese. Mix well.
- In a small bowl, prepare the vinaigrette. Whisk together the oils, lime juice and zest, Dijon mustard and basil.
- Adjust seasoning for the vinaigrette, then pour over salad. Mix well and serve.

Greek Salad

This salad is popular throughout the Mediterranean region and brings together health-giving ingredients that the ancient Minoans of Crete believed would assure long life.

Ingredients *(2 to 4 servings)*

1 small red onion, minced
1 cucumber, seeded, diced
2 large tomatoes, seeded, diced
8 to 10 black olives, pitted and sliced
¾ cup (180 ml) feta cheese, diced
3 tbsp (45 ml) olive oil
1 tbsp (15 ml) apple cider vinegar
½ tsp (2 ml) dried oregano
salt and pepper to taste

Instructions

- Combine diced vegetables, tomato and feta cheese in a large bowl.
- In a smaller bowl, prepare the vinaigrette by beating together the olive oil, vinegar, oregano and seasoning.
- Add vinaigrette to salad mixture and mix well. Serve garnished with a few whole black olives and a sprinkling of dried oregano.

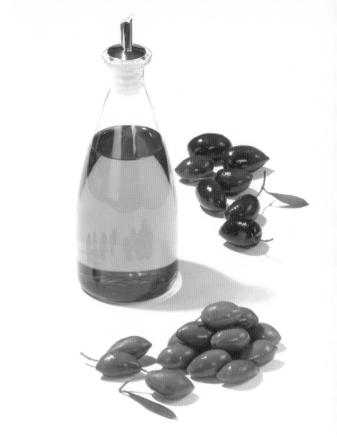

Sauces and Dips

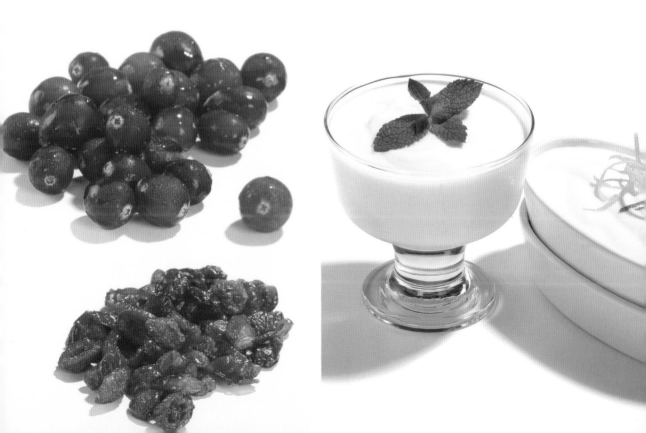

Sauces and Dips...
and Tasty Discoveries

What would a meat fondue be without all those great sauces? If the secret of a fine soup rests on the quality of the broth that enriches it, then the great flavor of a salad generally depends on the sauce or dressing it is topped with. Any simple combination of two or three vegetables changes in taste dramatically depending on whether it is served with a garlic vinaigrette, a lemony mayonnaise or a drizzling of curried cream sauce. Vinaigrettes, sauces and dips add style and elegance to a salad or a platter of crudités; they break the monotony and routine of a meal. Quite simply, they are the agents of great taste.

Sauces and Dips

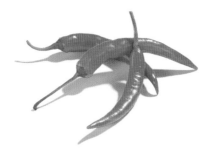

Aïoli Sauce

This simple, traditional sauce is originally from Provence and is a delicious way to enjoy all the health-giving benefits of raw garlic. You can vary the flavors simply by adding different fresh herbs such as basil, parsley or coriander (cilantro).

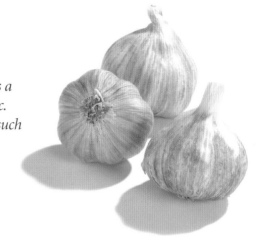

Ingredients *(2 servings)*

3 cloves of garlic
¼ cup (60 ml) olive oil
a little salt
1 tbsp (15 ml) lemon juice
1 egg yolk

Instructions

- Finely grind the garlic with a mortar and pestle, or mince the cloves very finely using a sharp knife or garlic press.

- Add the olive oil to the garlic, then add the salt, 1 tsp (5 ml) of lukewarm water and the lemon juice, mixing constantly.
- Stir in the egg yolk.
- Serve poured over raw or steamed vegetables (at room temperature).

Harissa Chili Sauce

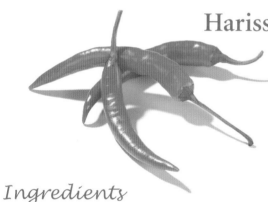

Although this North African (Maghrebian) hot sauce can only be used in small quantities, it contains compounds that relieve joint pain by stimulating the production of endorphins.

Instructions

- Wearing gloves, remove the seeds of the fresh chilies, or drain and pat dry the dried chilies before seeding. Put into a food processor.
- Add garlic, spices and salt, and mix at high speed.
- Add the oil in a thin stream, as for a mayonnaise, and continue to process.
- Transfer sauce to a small glass jar and add a bit more oil on top before closing. Will keep for at least six weeks in the refrigerator.

Ingredients

5 small, fresh hot chili peppers (or dried chilies soaked for 1 hour in hot water)
2 cloves of garlic, minced
2 tsp (10 ml) coriander seeds
2 tsp (10 ml) cumin seeds
2 tsp (10 ml) caraway seeds
a pinch of salt
½ cup (125 ml) olive oil

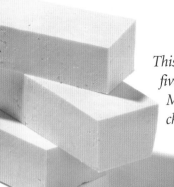

Tofu Mayonnaise

This multi-purpose sauce has the consistency of regular mayonnaise but contains five times less fat(!) To vary the flavor of this sauce, try adding curry paste or Mexican hot sauce. Also try adding aromatic herbs such as fresh basil, tarragon, chives or coriander (cilantro). It can be made into a vegetable dip by adding yogurt.

Instructions

- Mix together all the ingredients in a food processor.
- Season to taste and refrigerate.

Note

Since tofu is a food completely without flavor, the fine taste of this mayonnaise will depend on the quality of the olive oil used.

Ingredients

½ package (about 6 oz / 175 g) extra firm silken tofu
2 tbsp (30 ml) lemon juice
2 tbsp (30 ml) olive oil
2 tsp (10 ml) Dijon mustard
1 tsp (5 ml) honey
a few drops of Tabasco sauce
herbs and black pepper to taste

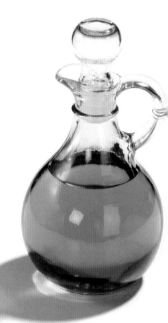

Egg-Free Light Mayonnaise

Of course the flavor of this sauce is not the same as real mayonnaise, but its consistency and appearance closely resemble its high-calorie cousin. This light mayonnaise becomes quite delicious when condiments or herbs are added.

Ingredients

3 tbsp (45 ml) unsweetened evaporated milk, refrigerated for a few hours
6 tbsp + 1 tsp (95 ml) olive oil
1 tsp (5 ml) Dijon mustard
juice of ½ lemon
3 tbsp (45 ml) olive oil

Instructions

- Beat the milk with the 6 tbsp + 1 tsp (95 ml) olive oil to obtain a smooth mixture.
- Add lemon juice, mustard, the 3 tbsp (45 ml) olive oil and beat again.
- Add flavorings of your choice (such as minced garlic, herbs or curry) to taste.

Tzatziki Sauce

This delicate, tangy sauce makes a light dip that accompanies grilled meats or fish. It is traditionally served in Greece as an hors-d'oeuvre with unleavened bread or pita.

Ingredients

1 cup (250 ml) plain yogurt
½ cucumber, seeded and chopped
2 cloves of garlic, minced
½ tsp (2 ml) fresh dill, chopped
1 tbsp (15 ml) olive oil
salt and pepper to taste

Instructions

- Line a sieve or strainer with two layers of cheese-cloth and place over a bowl. Pour yogurt into the cheesecloth and drain for a few hours in the refrigerator preferably overnight).
- Place the chopped cucumber in another sieve lined with cheesecloth and leave to drain for 1 hour.
- Press down to drain the liquid, then transfer cucumber to a small salad bowl.
- Add the drained yogurt, garlic, dill and olive oil. Mix well.
- Season with salt and pepper to taste.
- Cover and seal with plastic wrap and refrigerate for at least 2 hours before serving.

Cranberry Sauce with Orange and Ginger

This sauce is full of the powerful, health-giving antioxidants of the cranberry. It goes marvelously with roasted turkey, chicken or duck.

Ingredients

¾ lb (375 g) fresh cranberries
1 cup (250 ml) freshly squeezed orange juice
½ cup (125 ml) brown sugar
1 tbsp (15 ml) grated fresh ginger
½ tsp (1 ml) grated lemon zest

Instructions

- Mix the cranberries, orange juice, brown sugar, ginger and lemon zest in a saucepan.
- Bring to a boil, then lower the heat and let simmer for 15 minutes, stirring occasionally until the cranberries break open and the mixture thickens. Sauce will keep for at least a week in the refrigerator.

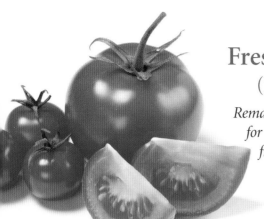

Fresh Tomato Sauce
(microwave recipe)

Remarkably simple to prepare, this delicious, versatile sauce is perfect for pasta dishes. It retains all the excellent health-giving benefits of fresh tomato and garlic.

Instructions

- Put olive oil, shallot and garlic in a microwave-safe dish and cook in microwave for 1 minute at the highest setting.
- Mix in tomatoes and cook for 5 minutes at the same setting.
- Add the basil, season to taste and cook for 1 more minute.
- Let sit for 3 minutes before serving.

Ingredients *(2 servings)*

2 tbsp (30 ml) olive oil
2 shallots, finely minced
1 clove of garlic, minced
4 fully ripe tomatoes, seeded and crushed
¼ cup (60 ml) finely chopped fresh basil or parsley
salt and pepper to taste

Curried Yogurt Dip
with Pineapple

The fine, tropical flavors of the pineapple and ginger in this appetizing, low-calorie dip combine wonderfully with the essence of the fresh coriander (cilantro).

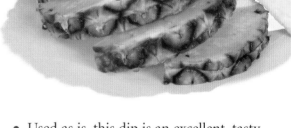

Ingredients

1 small container (about 6 oz / 180 g) plain yogurt
1 slice of pineapple, chopped
2 tbsp (30 ml) sesame seeds
1 tsp (5 ml) grated fresh ginger
½ tsp (2 ml) curry powder
2 bunches fresh coriander, finely chopped
salt and pepper to taste

- Used as is, this dip is an excellent, tasty vinaigrette for a sliced cabbage salad.
- The sauce can be thickened by adding 1 tbsp (15 ml) of mayonnaise or cream cheese.

Instructions

- Whisk together all the ingredients.

Blueberry Vinegar

Like cranberries, blueberries offer tremendous health-giving benefits. Try this elegant vinegar: a new use for this wonderful berry.

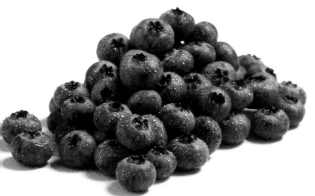

Ingredients

¾ cup (180 ml) fresh blueberries
apple cider vinegar (boiled) to cover the berries

Instructions

- Crush the blueberries and put them in a 1-cup (250-ml) glass jar. Fill the jar with the boiled apple cider vinegar, seal shut and let the blueberries macerate for 1 week, gently shaking the closed jar once or twice a day to mix.
- At the end of one week, strain the vinegar twice through a fine sieve to remove skins and seeds. Pour into a bottle. This vinegar will keep for at least a year.

Super-Healthy Vinaigrette

This salad dressing is made with several ingredients that are among the most health-giving foods known. Use this vinaigrette on a salad of sliced cabbage, delicate broccoli florets or crisp spinach leaves to make an appetizer positively bursting with healing properties that protect the body against disease.

Ingredients

¼ cup (60 ml) olive oil
2 tbsp (30 ml) apple cider vinegar
1 tsp (5 ml) honey
2 tbsp (30 ml) chopped fresh parsley (leaves and stems)
2 tbsp (30 ml) chopped fresh coriander (cilantro)
1 clove of garlic, minced
1 small shallot, chopped
½ tsp (2 ml) grated fresh ginger
a pinch of cayenne pepper
salt and pepper to taste

Instructions

- Place all ingredients in a blender or shaker. Mix for 1 minute.
- Use this vinaigrette on mixed lettuce leaves or other salad greens of your choice: Boston lettuce, roquette, curly chicory, Romaine lettuce, spinach, radicchio, arugula, etc.

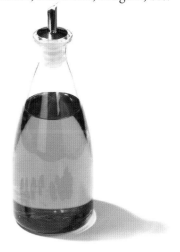

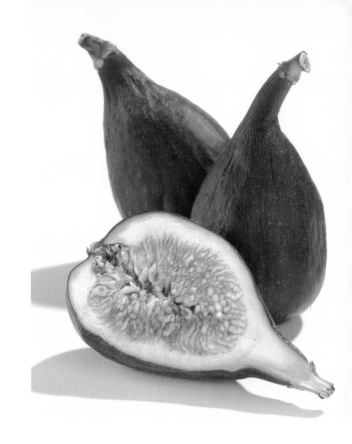

Desserts

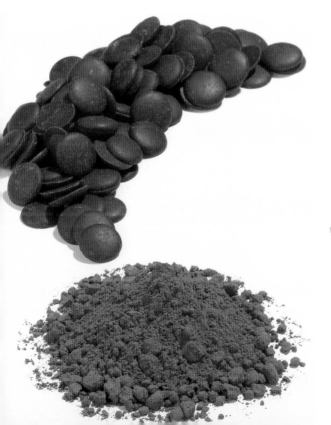

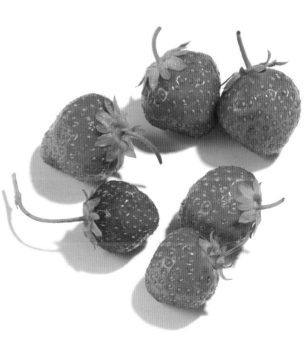

Desserts: The Finishing Touch

For most people, a fine meal is not complete without that sweet, finishing touch: dessert. The recipes included here follow our motto: healthy, simple and delicious. All of the desserts are full of healthy and health-giving foods, they are simple to prepare and, most of all, they are truly delicious. It is no accident that these desserts are well stocked with a variety of fruits. After all, fruits are a precious, nutritious gift from Mother Nature, full of essential vitamins and natural sugars that supply us with energy.

Dessert Recipes

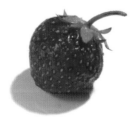

Bananas with Cinnamon and Rum

Here is a luscious, rich dessert that is quick to prepare and is best served after a light meal. If you replace the rum with rum extract and use yogurt instead of the whipped cream topping, the dessert will contain far fewer calories.

Ingredients *(4 servings)*

4 ripe bananas, cut in half, then sliced lengthwise
2 tbsp (30 ml) clarified butter (see page 152)
1 tsp (5 ml) ground cinnamon
5 tbsp (75 ml) rum or rum extract
3 tbsp (45 ml) honey
3 tbsp (45 ml) pecans

Instructions

- In a saucepan, sauté the banana slices in clarified butter for a few minutes. Remove from pan but keep warm.
- Pour rum into pan, add cinnamon and honey; heat until simmering, stirring until the sauce thickens somewhat.
- Roast the pecans in the oven at 350°F (180°C) for 5 minutes until golden. Chop coarsely.
- Add the nuts to the rum sauce and pour over the warm bananas.
- Serve with whipped cream or yogurt.

Blueberry Squares

These squares make a delicious snack. Blueberries help protect the eyes and combat "bad" (LDL) cholesterol.

Ingredients *(8 servings)*

½ cup (125 ml) walnuts or pecans, chopped
½ cup (125 ml) honey
2 cups (500 ml) whole wheat flour
½ cup (125 ml) non-hydrogenated margarine
2 cups (500 ml) fresh blueberries
2 eggs
½ tsp (2 ml) salt
1 ½ tsp (7 ml) ground cinnamon
6 tbsp (90 ml) wheat germ
1 tsp (5 ml) baking soda
1 tbsp (15 ml) apple cider vinegar
1 cup (250 ml) unsweetened evaporated milk

Instructions

- Preheat oven to 325°F (160°C).
- Spread a layer of chopped nuts on the bottom of a buttered 9 in. x 13 in. (22 x 32-cm) baking pan.
- Combine the honey, flour and margarine in a bowl.
- Transfer 2 cups (500 ml) of the mixture to the baking pan, spreading out evenly.
- Cover with the blueberries.
- In a bowl, beat the eggs with the cinnamon, wheat germ, baking soda, vinegar, evaporated milk and the rest of the flour mixture. Pour this mixture over the blueberries.
- Bake for about 35 minutes until edges are just golden.
- Allow to cool before cutting into squares.

Cranberry-Strawberry Purée

This fruit purée is especially recommended for people who suffer from frequent urinary tract or bladder infections.

Ingredients *(6 servings)*

¾ cup (180 ml) sugar
1 cup (250 ml) fresh strawberries
1 cup (250 ml) fresh cranberries
2 tbsp (30 ml) cranberry juice
2 tbsp (30 ml) cornstarch

Instructions

- In a saucepan, stir the sugar with ⅔ cup (150 ml) water to dissolve; bring to a boil.
- Add the berries and cranberry juice and let simmer gently for about 5 minutes.
- Dissolve the cornstarch into 2 tbsp (30 ml) of cold water, then add to the fruit mixture.
- Slowly bring to a boil, stirring constantly. Cook for 1 minute, continuing to stir.
- Let cool. Mix to smooth consistency in a blender.
- Serve over frozen yogurt.

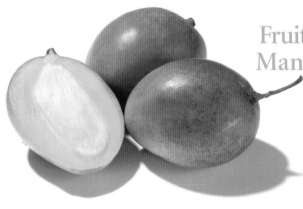

Fruit Cup with Mango Cream

Full of vitamins A and C, this luscious dessert is a favorite with children—and it is excellent for their growth.

Ingredients *(4 servings)*

2 kiwis, peeled and sliced
1 cup (250 ml) raspberries
2 tbsp (30 ml) orange juice
grated zest of 1 orange
1 ripe banana, sliced
1 large ripe mango, peeled, pitted and cut into bite-size pieces
½ cup (125 ml) whipping cream (35%)
fresh mint leaves for decoration

Instructions

- Put a mixture of the banana, kiwi and raspberries into 4 dessert bowls or fruit cups. Sprinkle with the orange juice and zest. Refrigerate for 30 minutes.
- Meanwhile, in a blender, purée the mango until smooth.
- With a hand-held mixer, whisk or egg-beater, beat the whipping cream until it forms stiff peaks.
- Gently add and blend mango purée into the whipped cream.
- Layer the mango cream over the fruit in each cup, decorate with mint leaves and serve chilled.

Crème Caramel with Coconut Milk

This healthy variation of the classic French dessert contains rich coconut cream and is a treat you'll certainly want to share with dinner guests.

Ingredients *(6 servings)*

¾ cup (180 ml) sugar
4 eggs
¼ cup (60 ml) sugar
1 tsp (5 ml) vanilla extract
14-oz (400-ml) can of coconut milk (or see page 247)
⅓ cup (75 ml) milk

Instructions

- Preheat oven to 325ºF (160ºC).
- In a saucepan, dissolve ¾ cup (180 ml) sugar into ¾ cup (180 ml) water, stirring while heating.
- Bring to a boil and let simmer without stirring, uncovered, until mixture turns caramel-colored.
- Let cool slightly and pour this caramel mixture into 6 small ramekins or oven-safe cups, each with a ½-cup (125 ml) capacity.
- In a bowl, beat together the eggs, remaining sugar and vanilla extract until well-blended.
- In a saucepan, heat the coconut milk and milk until just boiling (without letting it boil).
- Beat the hot coconut milk into the egg mixture.
- Divide mixture equally and carefully pour into the 6 ramekins. Place these in a large baking pan with enough boiling water to reach halfway up the sides.
- Bake for 40 minutes, or until the tops are firm to the touch.
- Remove ramekins from baking pan and let cool at room temperature.
- Cover and refrigerate.
- Just before serving, carefully turn over each ramekin on a serving dish to release the crème caramel.

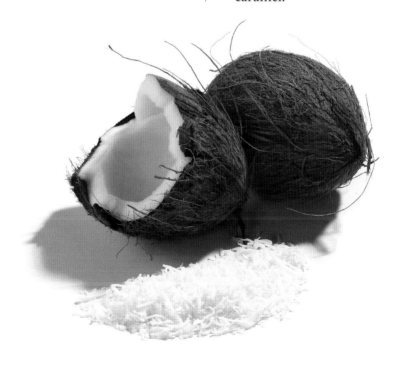

Curried Fruits

This warm, spicy-sweet fruit mixture makes for a delicious dessert that, topped with thickened yogurt, can also be an eye-opening breakfast dish.

Ingredients *(4 servings)*

⅓ cup (75 ml) brown sugar
1 tsp (5 ml) ground ginger
1 tsp (5 ml) cinnamon
½ tsp (2 ml) curry powder
¼ tsp (1 ml) nutmeg
¼ tsp (1 ml) ground cardamom
¼ tsp (1 ml) ground coriander
¼ cup (60 ml) orange juice
¼ cup (60 ml) rum or rum extract
2 tbsp (30 ml) lemon juice
2 apples, cored and cubed
2 peaches, pitted and cubed
2 pears, cored and cubed
1 cup (250 ml) strawberries or raspberries
1 banana, sliced

Instructions

- Mix together the brown sugar, spices and orange juice in a large saucepan. Cook for a few minutes until sugar is melted and turns syrupy.
- Add the rum or rum extract and lemon juice; bring to a boil.
- Add apple, peach and pear to the syrup mixture and cook for a few minutes until the fruits are tender.
- Add the strawberries or raspberries and the banana. Reheat and serve.

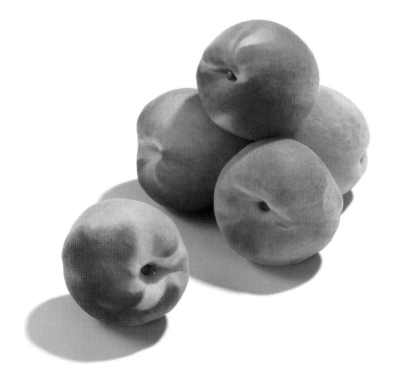

Zucchini Chocolate Loaf Cake

Thanks to the zucchini, this cake is soft and moist without being overly rich: a delicious, light chocolate cake with fiber and other health-giving nutrients.

Ingredients

½ cup (125 ml) unsweetened cocoa powder
1 cup (250 ml) all-purpose flour
½ cup (125 ml) buckwheat flour
¼ tsp (1 ml) baking powder
½ tsp (2 ml) baking soda
½ tsp (2 ml) salt
2 eggs
1 cup (250 ml) sugar
¾ cup (180 ml) grapeseed or sunflower oil
1 ½ cups (375 ml) grated zucchini (2 medium zucchinis)
grated zest of 1 orange
½ cup (125 ml) walnuts or pecans, chopped

Instructions

- Preheat oven to 350ºF (180ºC).
- In a large bowl, sift together the dry ingredients: cocoa powder, flours, baking powder, baking soda and salt.
- In a second bowl, beat the eggs. Add sugar and beat again. Add grapeseed oil, then zucchini and orange zest.
- Add to this mixture the dry ingredients, a spoonful at a time, mixing well after each. Add the nuts and mix again.
- Pour batter into an oiled or greased loaf pan.
- Bake for 75 minutes, or until a toothpick inserted into the center comes out clean.
- Let cool before icing with Dairy-Free Chocolate Icing (see below).

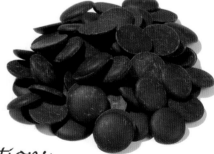

Dairy-Free Chocolate Icing

Ingredients

2 oz (60 g) bittersweet chocolate
2 tbsp (30 ml) butter or non-hydrogenated margarine
1 tbsp (15 ml) honey

Instructions

- In a double boiler (or Pyrex bowl sitting over a saucepan of boiling water), slowly melt the chocolate with the butter or margarine. Stir in the honey, then let cool to room temperature before icing your cake.

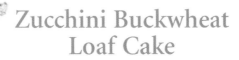

Zucchini Buckwheat Loaf Cake

Similar to carrot cake, this zucchini cake is just as rich and flavorful, with the added health benefits of the buckwheat, a grain that improves circulation and lowers high blood pressure.

Ingredients

2 eggs, beaten
¾ cup (180 ml) sugar
½ cup (125 ml) grapeseed or sunflower oil
2 medium zucchinis, unpeeled, grated
¾ cup (180 ml) whole wheat flour
½ cup (125 ml) buckwheat flour
¾ tsp (4 ml) baking powder
½ tsp (2 ml) baking soda
¾ tsp (4 ml) cinnamon
½ tsp (2 ml) nutmeg
½ tsp (2 ml) salt
grated zest of 1 orange
½ cup (125 ml) chopped pecans or walnuts

Instructions

- Preheat oven to 350°F (180°C).
- Grease a loaf pan with butter or oil.
- Beat together the eggs, sugar, oil and grated zucchini in a bowl.
- In a second bowl, sift together the remaining ingredients, except for the nuts. Add to the zucchini mixture, one spoonful at a time, mixing after each addition.
- Add the nuts and mix well.
- Carefully spoon the batter into the lined loaf pan.
- Bake for 1 to 1 ¼ hours or until a toothpick inserted into the center comes out clean.
- Let cool before removing from pan.
- Keep cake refrigerated until ready to add icing (see below and page 237).

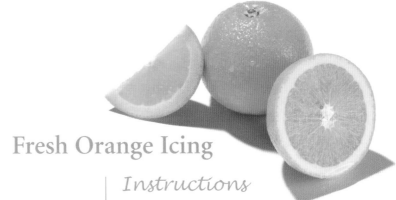

Fresh Orange Icing

Ingredients

1 ⅓ cup (325 ml) icing sugar
¼ cup (60 ml) non-hydrogenated margarine
grated zest of 1 orange
1 tbsp (15 ml) orange juice (or slightly more)

Instructions

- Blend margarine and icing sugar thoroughly.
- Stir in orange zest, then add orange juice a drop at a time, beating well between additions to obtain a spreadable consistency.

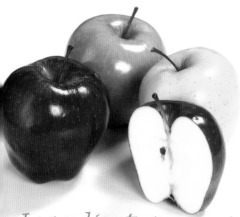

Home-Style Baked Apples

Served after a meal, these old-fashioned baked apples are delicious. They are also a tasty addition alongside roast pork or chicken.

Instructions

- Preheat oven to 375ºF (190ºC).
- Arrange the apples on a buttered baking sheet.
- Mix margarine with brown sugar, rolled oats, orange zest and juice, cinnamon and nuts.
- Fill the 4 apples with the mixture.
- Bake for 30 minutes, or until apples are softened.

* Remove cores with a corer or a small paring knife. Also remove a few thin bands of apple peel with a peeler.

Ingredients *(4 servings)*

4 cooking apples (e.g. Cortland), washed and kept whole, with core removed*
2 tbsp (30 ml) non-hydrogenated margarine
¼ cup (60 ml) brown sugar
¼ cup (60 ml) rolled oats or spelt flakes
juice and grated zest of half an orange
1 tsp (5 ml) cinnamon
¼ cup (60 ml) chopped walnuts, pecans or hazelnuts

Warm Fig and Apricot Fruit Compote

This is a wintertime dessert par excellence that furnishes the body with energy and fiber—a protection against cardiovascular disease.

Ingredients *(4 servings)*

¾ cup (180 ml) dried figs
1 cup (250 ml) dried apricots
½ cup (125 ml) raisins
¼ cup (60 ml) dried apples
¼ cup (60 ml) brown sugar, packed
½ cup (125 ml) almonds, chopped
¼ cup (60 ml) butter or non-hydrogenated margarine, melted
2 tbsp (30 ml) dark rum
1 tsp (5 ml) grated lemon zest
1 tsp (5 ml) lemon juice
1 tsp (5 ml) cinnamon

Instructions

- In a large saucepan, cover the dried figs, apricots, raisins and apples with water.
- Bring to a boil over medium heat and let simmer, uncovered, for 15 minutes.
- Drain the fruits, let cool, then chop.
- Return fruits to the saucepan and add remaining ingredients.
- Bring to a boil over medium heat and let simmer, covered this time, for 5 minutes.
- Serve over frozen yogurt.

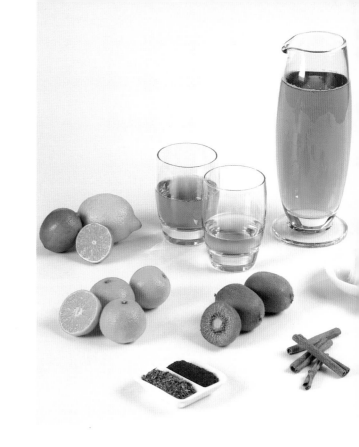

Beverages
and Other
Preparations

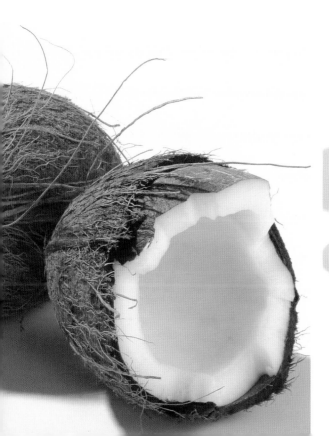

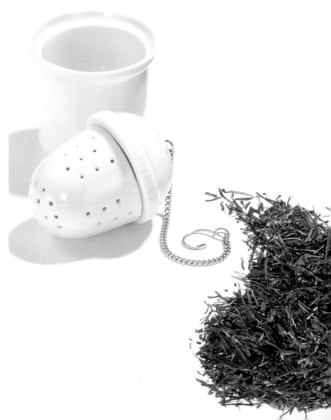

Beverages: Healing Tonics, Hot and Cold

With the help of a reliable juicer you can quickly prepare an almost infinite variety of fruit and vegetable juices that will allow you to take full advantage of all the goodness and health-giving properties these foods have to offer. The following beverage suggestions do not require a juicer, all of them are naturally thirst-quenching and together they offer a wide array of healing properties.

Beverages and Other Preparations

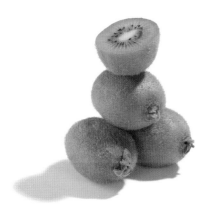

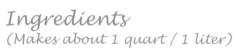

Ginger Beer

Ginger ale and most other ginger drinks sold at supermarkets are full of added sugar and coloring and do not retain any of the extra-ordinary health-giving benefits of ginger. So here is a never-fail recipe for a refreshing drink with all of the root's curative properties.

Ingredients
(Makes about 1 quart / 1 liter)

¾ cup (180 ml) fresh ginger root, peeled, coarsely chopped into ½-in (1-cm) pieces
4 cups (1 liter) water
2 tbsp (30 ml) honey

Instructions

- Bring the water to a boil in a large saucepan and add the chopped ginger.
- Cover, lower heat and let simmer for 30 minutes.
- Filter liquid, stir in honey, let cool; then refrigerate.
- To serve cold, add one part ginger drink to three parts carbonated mineral water.

Summertime Kiwi Smoothie

Here is a summer drink bursting with flavor—and vitamin C.

Ingredients *(4 servings)*

4 ripe kiwis, peeled
4 ice cubes
½ cup + 2 tbsp (155 ml) pineapple juice

Instructions

- In a blender, mix together all of the ingredients. Serve with slices of orange or lemon.

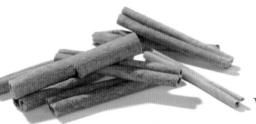

Hot Cider with Cinnamon

This simple, heartwarming drink is an excellent wintertime apéritif.

Ingredients *(2 servings)*

2 cups (500 ml) apple cider (or apple juice)
3 cinnamon sticks

Instructions

- Pour the cider, or for a non-alcoholic version, apple juice, into a saucepan. Add cinnamon sticks and heat gently. Serve.

Sparkling Lemonade

This wonderfully thirst-quenching drink offers cancer-fighting antioxidants in the form of a healthy dose of vitamin C.

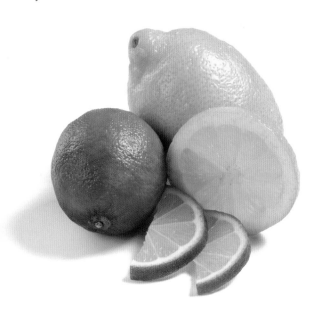

Ingredients *(4 servings)*

1 lime
2 lemons
3 clementines
¼ cup (60 ml) honey
3 cups (750 ml) carbonated mineral water

Instructions

- Squeeze fruits to obtain about 1 cup (250 ml) of juice. Squeeze 1 or 2 more fruits of your choice if necessary.
- Filter the juice and pour into a glass jar or jug. Add honey and stir well. Refrigerate.
- Pour mineral water into the jar or jug, then serve in glasses decorated with fruit slices and mint leaves.

Green Tea with Ginger and Mint

With its elegant aromas, this infusion aids digestion and helps to soothe the nerves.

Ingredients *(2 servings)*

1 to 2 tsp (5 to 10 ml) green tea
1 to 2 tsp (5 to 10 ml) fresh spearmint leaves
1 piece of ginger root, peeled
2 cups (500 ml) boiling water

Instructions

- Boil the water. Use some hot water to heat the teapot.
- Drop green tea, mint leaves and ginger into teapot.
- Add boiling water to tea and let steep for 5 minutes before serving.

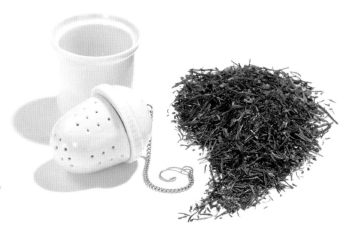

Coconut Milk

This mixture is used in Thai cooking and other Southeast Asian recipes calling for coconut milk.

Ingredients *(4 servings)*

1 ½ cups (375 ml) unsweetened coconut flakes
1 cup (250 ml) boiling water

Instructions

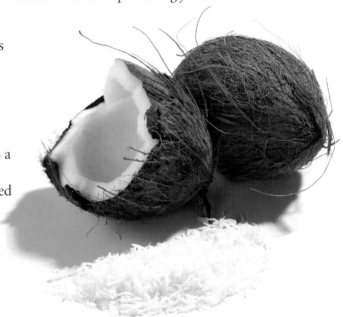

- Place coconut flakes in a blender. Pour the boiling water over the coconut.
- Activate blender for a few seconds to mix to a fine consistency. Let sit for 30 minutes.
- Filter the coconut liquid through a sieve lined with cheesecloth placed over a bowl, pressing down slightly to remove all the liquid.
- Store in a sealed jar in the refrigerator.

Almond (or Walnut) Butter

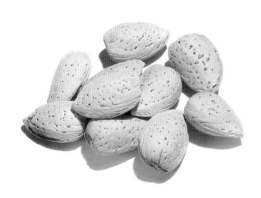

Ingredients

½ cup (125 ml) unsalted almonds (or walnuts)
2 tbsp (30 ml) sunflower or grapeseed oil

Instructions

- Put the almonds (or walnuts) in a blender and grind to a fine consistency.
- Add the oil, a teaspoon at a time, mixing with each addition until a thick peanut butter-like consistency is achieved.
- Transfer to a sealed jar and store in the refrigerator.

Spice Mixtures

To add the most authentic flavors and aromas to your recipes, it is best to make your own spice mixtures. This can be done by grinding grains in a mortar or in a small electric coffee grinder reserved for this purpose. (You don't want to flavor your spices with coffee—or vice versa!) Once whole spices and seeds are ground and mixed together, transfer them to well-labeled glass jars and store in a cupboard out of the light. Spice mixtures will continue to develop in the jar and will reach the peak of their flavors in the first few weeks. For this reason it is best to prepare small quantities of spice mixtures at a time.

Indian Curry Spice

1 tsp (5 ml) cumin
1 tsp (5 ml) coriander
½ tsp (2 ml) fenugreek
½ tsp (2 ml) turmeric
1 ½ tsp (7 ml) black pepper
¼ tsp (1 ml) cardamom
1 tsp (5 ml) chili powder

Maghrebian (North African) Spice

1 tsp (5 ml) cumin
1 tsp (5 ml) fennel seed
1 tsp (5 ml) dried basil
1 tsp (5 ml) dried mint

Cajun Spice

1 tsp (5 ml) cayenne pepper
1 tsp (5 ml) crushed chili peppers
2 tsp (10 ml) paprika
1 tsp (5 ml) oregano
1 tsp (5 ml) thyme
1 tsp (5 ml) fennel seed

Mixed Italian Herbs

1 tsp (5 ml) rosemary
1 tsp (5 ml) dried basil
2 tsp (10 ml) savory
2 tsp (10 ml) marjoram

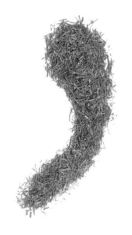

Appendices

The three useful tables beginning on this page summarize for you which healing foods are associated with which health conditions or diseases. Also included is a list of foods to be avoided if you have certain health conditions, as well as a list of foods certain groups of people should avoid.

Foods recommended for specific health problems

Health problem	*Recommended foods*
Aging (deterioration) of cells	avocado, mango, orange, raspberry
Allergies	fenugreek
Alzheimer's disease	pear, sweet potato, turmeric
Anemia	apricot, beet, cantaloupe, carrot, cress, eggplant fenugreek, lemon, parsley, seaweed, spinach
Anorexia	fennel, onion
Appendicitis	tomato
Arrhythmia (cardiac)	'fatty' fish
Arteriosclerosis (hardening of the arteries)	pineapple, rye
Arthritis	cabbage, cherry, 'fatty' fish, flaxseed, garlic, ginger, lettuce, orange, turmeric
Arthrosis (joint afflictions)	cantaloupe, celery, fenugreek, pineapple, turmeric
Asthma	squash, orange
Atherosclerosis (a type of hardening of arteries)	onion, tea
Bacterial infection	green bean, carrot, garlic, honey, leek, orange, seaweed, tea, yogurt
Bladder infection	apple cider vinegar
Bronchitis	fenugreek, onion
Bronchitis, chronic	chili pepper
Cancer (*see also specific types listed below*)	asparagus, barley, blueberry, broccoli, cantaloupe, celery, chili pepper, corn, garlic, grape (and red wine), grapefruit, kiwi, lettuce, mango, onion, orange, parsley, pea, pineapple, potato, (black and red) radish, spinach, sweet potato, tangerine, tea, walnut, wheat germ, zucchini
Cancer, breast	cauliflower, flaxseed, 'fatty' fish, olives (and olive oil), rice, soy, tomato
Cancer, colon	cabbage, cauliflower, 'fatty' fish, fig, flaxseed, parsnip, pear, rice, rutabaga, tomato, turnip
Cancer, endometrial	squash, tomato
Cancer, liver	apricot

Health problem	Recommended foods
Cancer, lung	apricot, tomato
Cancer, pancreatic	apricot
Cancer, prostate	cauliflower, flaxseed, rice, soy, tomato
Cancer, rectal	turnip
Cancer, skin	apricot, turmeric
Cancer, stomach	cabbage, tomato
Cancer, uterine	flaxseed
Cardiac (heart) afflictions	spinach, squash
Cardiovascular disease	apple, (dried) beans, broccoli, cherry, chili pepper, coconut, cress, 'fatty' fish, flaxseed, leek, lettuce, mango, nuts, oats, olive oil, papaya, parsnip, peach, (sweet red) pepper, raspberry, (brown) rice, rye, walnut, wheat germ, (red) wine, soybean,
Cataract	broccoli, cabbage, cantaloupe, sweet pepper, tomato, turmeric
Cholesterol	apple, artichoke, asparagus, avocado, banana, barley, carrot, chili pepper, corn, eggplant, fenugreek, fig, flaxseed, grape (and red wine), grapefruit, kiwi, (shiitake) mushroom, nuts, oats, olives and olive oil, onions, pea, pear, plantain, plum and prune, rice, seaweed, soy, spinach, sweet pepper, walnut
Chronic fatigue	apple cider vinegar
Circulatory (blood) problems	buckwheat
Coagulation (blood thickening)	red chili pepper, onion
Common cold	cabbage, cauliflower, clementine, fenugreek, ginger, grapefruit, honey, kiwi, lemon, peas, pineapple
Congenital malformation, prevention of	beet
Congestion of the lungs	red chili pepper
Constipation	avocado, barley, carrot, fig, honey, plum and prune, squash, strawberry
Cough	barley, black radish
Cramps (stomach) and colic	fennel
Cystitis (urinary tract infection)	cranberry
Degenerative diseases	blueberry
Dental cavities	apple, corn, grape, tea
Depression	apricot, 'fatty' fish, flaxseed, spinach
Diabetes	blueberry, fenugreek, oats, onion, sweet potato
Diarrhea	apple, apricot, banana, blueberry, carrot, rice, tea, turmeric, walnut
Digestion problems	buckwheat, papaya, parsnip, plum and prune, tea
Equilibrium, nervous	banana

Health problem	Recommended foods
Eye infection	cranberry
Eyesight, problems with	blueberry, cranberry
Fatigue, chronic	apple cider vinegar
Flatulence	fennel, ginger, parsley
Flu, see *Influenza*	
Gallstones	millet
Gastroenteritis	apple cider vinegar, yogurt
Gout	cantaloupe, cherry, endive, lemon, lettuce, strawberry
Headache related to indigestion	apple cider vinegar
Headache	ginger
Heartburn (stomach irritation)	pineapple
Hemorrhage	buckwheat, grapefruit, orange
Hemorrhoids	apple cider vinegar, grape, plantain, squash
Herpes zoster (shingles)	cabbage
High blood pressure	avocado, red chili pepper
HIV (Human Immunodeficiency Virus)	avocado, shiitake mushroom, strawberry, yogurt
Hypertension (see also *High blood pressure*)	apple cider vinegar, banana, buckwheat, cantaloupe, celery, chili pepper, fenugreek, fig, garlic, grape (and red wine), Jerusalem, artichoke, kiwi, lettuce, olive oil, potato, (brown) rice, rye, tea
Indigestion and digestive problems	artichoke, avocado, pineapple, (black) radish
Indigestion and digestive problems (prevention)	celery, ginger, wheat germ
Inflammation, joint (see also *Arthrosis*)	turmeric
Inflammation, mouth (oral)	blueberry, plantain, raspberry
Inflammation, respiratory tract	chili pepper, fennel, onion, plantain
Inflammation, skin	plantain
Inflammation, various	pineapple
Influenza	beet, cauliflower, ginger, honey
Insomnia	apricot, grapefruit
Intestinal gas, see *Flatulence*	
Intestinal irritation	fig
Irritable Bowel Syndrome	artichoke
Itching, various	apple cider vinegar
Kidney ailments	brown rice
Kidney infection	apple cider vinegar
Lung conditions	squash
Menopausal malaise	soybean
Menstrual malaise	millet, parsley
Motion sickness	ginger
Nausea	ginger
Neuralgia (nerve pain)	fenugreek

Obesity	sarrasin
Osteoporosis	flaxseed
Rheumatism	cabbage, cantaloupe, celeriac, celery, cherry, eggplant, ginger, lettuce, parsnip, potato, raspberry, seaweed
Shingles, see *Herpes zoster*	
Skin conditions	turmeric
Skin disease	mango, turmeric
Sore throat	apple cider vinegar, barley, honey, pineapple
Stomach pain	cinnamon, garlic, lemon, raspberry
Tumor	fig, mushroom (shiitake), seaweed
Ulcer	cabbage, ginger, honey, potato, yogurt
Urinary disease, see *Cystitis*	
Urinary infection	raspberry
Varicose veins	cabbage, red grape
Venous insufficiency	blueberry, grape
Viral infection	cabbage, garlic, grape, mushroom (shiitake), tea
Vomiting	ginger
Worms (parasitic)	fenugreek, garlic, lemon, parsley, turmeric

Foods to be <u>avoided</u> according to specific health problems

Health problem	*Foods to avoid*
Allergies, various (see also specific allergies)	apple cider vinegar, peanut, strawberry, tomato, walnut, wheat germ
Aspirin allergy	apricot, tomato
Asthma	apricot
Bile duct blockage	artichoke
Constipation	mache (corn salad lettuce)
Cystitis (urinary tract infection)	asparagus
Diabetes	banana, beet, cantaloupe, cranberry, dandelion greens, potato
Diarrhea	olive oil
Diverticulitis (intestinal inflammation)	flaxseed
Dyspepsia (indigestion)	cantaloupe, cherry
Enteritis	cantaloupe
Flatulence (intestinal gas)	(dried) beans, cauliflower, leek, turnip
Gastric (stomach) irritations	garlic, turmeric
Gluten intolerance (celiac disease)	barley, oats, rye, strawberry, wheat
Gout	asparagus, cauliflower, dandelion greens
Heartburn (stomach indigestion)	tomato

Health problem	Foods to avoid
Hypertension (high blood pressure)	plantain, seaweed, wheat germ
Intestinal irritations	raspberry
Irritable Bowel Syndrome	corn
Jaundice	chicory
Lethargy (digestive)	turnip
Low-sodium diet	celeriac, celery, olive
Migraine headache	onion, green tomato
Mouth irritations	mango (unpeeled), orange
Oral Allergy Syndrome	cherry, kiwi, orange, peach, zucchini, or any fruits or vegetables provoking an itching in the lips, mouth and throat
Ovarian cancer	flaxseed
Parasites (intestinal)	raw fish
Rheumatism	asparagus, dandelion greens
Sensitive stomach	(red) chili pepper, cress, papaya, radish, (green) sweet pepper
Skin conditions and irritations	parsnip, strawberry
Stomach pain	apple cider vinegar
Stomach ulcer	turmeric
Thyroid condition	black radish
Urinary tract infection, susceptibility to	spinach

Group at risk	Foods to avoid
Children	tea
Nursing mothers	tea
Pregnant women	fenugreek, ginger, parsley, tea
Breast-feeding infants	honey
Persons susceptible to weight gain	avocado, banana, coconut, fig, walnut
Persons sensitive to mold and mildew	soybean
Persons susceptible to hemorrhaging	olive

Conversion Tables

Cooking Temperatures

Fahrenheit	Celsius	Microwave Setting	Thermostat
150	70	1	very low – min
170	80	2	low
200	100	3	low
250	120	3	low
275	140	4	low
300	150	4	low
325	160	5	medium
350	180	5	medium
375	190	6	medium
400	200	6	medium
425	220	7	medium-high
450	230	7	medium-high
475	240	8	high
500	260	8	high
525	270	9	very high
550	290	9	very high-max

Weights and Measures

Imperial weights (ounce / pound)	Metric weight (gram / kilogram)
½ ounce (oz)	15 g
1 oz	30 g
2 oz	60 g
3 oz	90 g
4 oz (¼ pound / lb)	125 g (113.5 g)
6 oz	187.5 g
8 oz (½ lb)	250 g (227 g)
12 oz (¾ lb)	375 g
16 oz (1 lb)	500 g (454 g)
24 oz (1 ½ lb)	750 g
32 oz (2 lb)	1,000 g (1 kg)
3 lb	1,500 g (1.5 kg)
4 lb	2,000 g (2 kg)

Weights and Measures *(continued)*

Liquid measure (fluid ounces)	Cups (tablespoons)	Metric (milliliters)
1 fl oz	⅛ cup (2 tbsp)	30 ml
2 fl oz	⅓ cup (4 tbsp)	60 ml
2.5 fl oz	¼ cup (5 tbsp)	75 ml
3 fl oz	⅜ cup	100 ml
4 fl oz	½ cup	125 ml
5 fl oz	⅝ cup	160 ml
6 fl oz	¾ cup	180 ml
7 fl oz	⅞ cup	220 ml
8 fl oz	1 cup	250 ml
10 fl oz	1 ¼ cups	300 ml
12 fl oz	1 ½ cups	375 ml
14 fl oz	1 ¾ cups	430 ml
16 fl oz	2 cups	500 ml
20 fl oz	2 ½ cups	625 ml

Glossary

ANTIANEMIC
A substance taken to treat patients with anemia to increase their levels of hemoglobin and / or red blood cell count.

ANTIOXIDANT
A compound found primarily in fruits and vegetables that slows or inhibits the oxidation processes and the damaging effects of free radicals which contribute to the deterioration and aging of the body's cells.

ANTIBIOTIC / ANTIBACTERIAL
A substance that destroys bacteria.

ANTISEPTIC
A substance that stops or inhibits the decay of tissues by slowing or stopping infection by micro-organisms such as bacteria.

ANTISPASMODIC
A substance that diminishes contractions, cramps and convulsions.

ANTIVIRAL
A substance that works to combat and destroy viruses.

BETA CAROTENE
An antioxidant compound that is also a pigment, giving certain fruits and vegetables a rich orange-red color (such as apricot, carrot, cantaloupe and red pepper).

DEPURANT
That which helps to purify the body by promoting the removal of waste.

DIURETIC
That which helps the cleansing of the body by stimulating the excretion of liquids via the urinary tract.

EXPECTORANT
A medication that promotes the expulsion of mucus secretions in the air passages.

FOLATE *OR* FOLIC ACID
A molecule that interacts with vitamin B_{12} in the production of DNA and RNA—important compounds in the growth of the body's cells, including red blood cells.

HYPOCHOLESTEREMIANT
A substance that lowers blood cholesterol.

HYPOTENSOR
A substance that lowers blood pressure.

IMMUNOSTIMULANT
A substance that amplifies or increases the function of the immune system and formation of antibodies.

MONOUNSATURATED FATS
Fatty acids that lower the levels of 'bad' (LDL) cholesterol in the body and play a beneficial role in protecting against cardiovascular disease and narrowing of the arteries.

TRACE ELEMENTS
Chemical elements that are needed in small amounts for the maintenance of good health.

REMINERALISATION
The restoration of minerals needed by the body, especially in the bones.

STOMACHIC
A substance that is beneficial to the stomach or stimulates and improves digestion in the stomach.

VERMIFUGE (OR ANTHELMINTIC)
That which provokes or promotes the expulsion of parasitic worms from the intestines.

Index of Foods

Index of Recipes

Table of Contents